FOOD THERAPY FOR SELF CURE

Gina Yang

My deepest thanks and love to the Universe for the wonderful guidance to bring this book to the earth for healing. My thanks and love to my dearly beloved women in my life grandma, and nanny, and the people who generously shared their treasures and experiences. My love and thanks to those who helped me to bring this book to this world in a physical form.

Contents

Preface

Every person must experience birth, aging, illness and death but suffering is not the purpose for us came to this world. Every life time is for us to experience, to learn, and to gain our freedom, free from all human limitations. The purpose of this book is to help you to free yourself from the illness, the prescription drugs, the unnecessary surgeries, and the medical cost. In this book in addition to food remedies you also can find interesting stories, health-related information, real cases, and detailed explanations of how to use food therapy for self-healing in every chapter.

Currently the development of medicine and extensive application of chemical drugs bring many drug-induced diseases. It has become a common aspiration of people to seek alternative medicine that is free of toxins and side effects. Can food replace chemical drugs to cure diseases? After you finish this book you will realize foods are not just to meet our most basic survival needs they are also play an important role in healing ailments. From this book you shall discover that many foods are listed in classic Chinese herbal medicine books as herbs. Food therapy always plays an important role in traditional Chinese medicine. In fact in any culture there was a time when people only relied on natural remedies for healing. One purpose of this book is to raise people's awareness of not overly rely on doctors, surgeries, and prescription drugs. Every person should take responsibility for his or her own health. Almost all health issues which doctors believe are incurable you can find cure in this book. You have free will to decide to rely on doctors or use your own power to overcome the disease.

In my practice I have seen many health issues are caused by misleading health care education regarding to the diseases, healthy diet, vitamins and supplements. For that reason in addition to food remedies this book also includes the explanation of the functions of human body and the cause of the diseases based on Traditional Chinese medicine theory. Since most remedies in this book are based on the theory of Chinese medicine at the beginning I would like to help my readers know a little bit of traditional Chinese medicine. With this information you shall have more confidence on your journey of self healing. I have no intention of opposing Western medicine. Chinese medicine and Western medicine are two completely different medical systems. We cannot judge them or compare them to each other with good or bad. Like a Chinese medicine doctor said we do not compare Chinese medical system with Western medical system just like we do not compare green tea with coffee, or compare Chinese painting with western oil painting. However, **traditional Chinese medicine is a complete and advanced medical system, Western medicine is not.** Why I dare to make this statement? Because Western medical system is developed by humans and there are still a lot of unknowns in Western medical studies. For most diseases there is no cure in Western medical practice. The development of Western medicine started from the studies of anatomy and physiology, therefore their studies are limited to visible and physical level of a human body. For this reason the cause of most diseases remains unknown to Western medicine. Today the knowledge of anatomy and physiology combine with advanced technology give Western medicine the advantage in diagnosis and in cases of emergency. For acute problems or serious injuries Western medicine is a good choice.

Chinese medicine is not developed by Chinese people. The knowledge of traditional Chinese medicine was passed down to Chinese people from advanced life (ascended beings). Traditional Chinese medicine is part of the great ancient wisdom that is older than human history. This profound knowledge goes beyond the limits of our human dimension by connecting our human perceptions with the nature and the Universe. This medical system is so complete it includes diagnosis, treatment, prognosis, and prevention of diseases. The detailed theory about human body includes the physical and the intangible. The intangible part of a human body includes energy, function of the organic system, emotion, and mind. The theory of Chinese medicine has precise explanations about both visible and invisible parts of a human body. These days with the most advanced technology the energy in a human body is still invisible to human eyes but the charts of Jingluo which is the energy passageway within a human body have been used in Chinese medicine for thousands of years. Ancient Buddhist teachings tell us that a human body is a small universe and that 99% of the universe is invisible to our physical eyes so is a human body. Chinese medicine is energy medicine. The core of Chinese medicine is "Qi" (energy) an Intangible and invisible part of a human body. What is Chinese medicine? Most people will say "acupuncture". Acupuncture is only one treatment in Chinese medicine practice.

There are three levels of the practice in traditional Chinese medicine. The highest level of Chinese medicine is taught and practiced by those who are seeking or have found the truth of the Universe and life. The purpose of this level of practice is for an individual to achieve the greatest human potential and reach the maximum level of enlightenment. This kind of teaching was kept in secret in the past and passed down only from a master to the one who is ready to receive the knowledge by the word of mouth. The herbs are used at this level of Chinese medicine is for purify the physical body, maintain youth and beauty, prolong life, and even overcome death. Those who practice Chinese medicine at this level are not doctors. They are the masters of life.

The second level practice of Chinese medicine focus on prevention of diseases and maintain good health. Therapeutic exercises, such as Taiji, Yoga, and meditation, etc., food therapy, and healthy life style belong to this level of Chinese medicine.

The lowest level practice of Chinese medicine is to treat diseases. Today's health care practices all belong to this level of medicine. The treatment in traditional Chinese medicine is so down-to-earth, a well-trained Chinese medicine practitioner does not rely on any equipment or lab work to do diagnosis. From the visible he can see the invisible. There are no surgeries performed in Chinese medicine practice. All treatment is natural, safe and performed on the surface of the body even for treating internal diseases. Acupuncture needles are the only medical waste in Chinese medicine practice. Chinese herbal remedies are safe, effective, and affordable.

The first Chinese herbal medicine book called "Shen Nong Ben Cao" was written at a very ancient time. According to historical records, the author Shen Nong was not an ordinary human. Neither does he like a human. His name Shen Nong means divine farmer. It is said to help Chinese people to survive on this planet, Shen Nong came to earth. After he tasted all the plants and was poisoned seventy times he completed the book that taught Chinese people the properties of each plant and what kinds of plants can be eaten as food, and what kinds of plants can be used as herbs to treat ailments. This book is the foundation of Chinese herbal medicine.

Another very important Chinese herbal remedies book was written by a famous Chinese medicine doctor 2500 years ago. The book's name is called "Qian Jin Fang" that means "the remedies that worth thousands of gold". The doctor's name is Simiao Sun. When he was young he lived in a Taoist monastery and was proficient in astronomy and medicine. One day when he was collecting herbs in the mountain he saw a small black snake wounded by a cowboy. He used herbs to attend the snake's wound and put it back into the mountain. Ten days later when Simiao Sun was walking in the street, a young man dressed in all white riding a white horse came up to him, dismounted and fell to his knees and said "Thank you for saving my brother's life." Before Simiao Sun realize what was happening the young man invited him to see his father and helped him get on the horse. The young man led the horse and walked very quickly. Soon they came to a city with brilliant palace. A man looking like a king, followed by many attendants, came to meet him and said "I am deeply grateful for master's mercy and deliberately had my son go for you." Then pointing to a little boy, dressed in black standing next to him, he said, "Ten days ago this child went out alone and was wounded by a cowboy. Luckily you saved his life." The King let the child bow to the master. At this moment Simiao Sun realized the boy was the black snake he saved ten days ago. He quietly asked an attendant, "What is this place?" and was told the place is "Jing Yang Shui Fu", which was well known by Chinese people as dragon's palace. The King set a banquet to entertain Simiao Sun. Simiao Sun was practicing Taoist fasting so he only had a little wine. After spending three days at the dragon's palace Simiao Sun wanted to return. The King offered him a lot of gold and silver as a gift but Simiao Sun refused to take them, so the King had his son brought a book called "Long Gong Qi Fang". The book's name means magic remedies of dragon's palace, it contains thirty herbal remedies. Simiao Sun accepted the book. He used those remedies to treat his patients and found the results are very efficacious. Later he added these remedies in his own collection and wrote a herbal medicine book "Qian Jin Fang" which has been used by Chinese medicine doctors to this day.

Simiao Sun lived more than 100 years. All his life he used Chinese medicine to help working people and save lives. One day he took a bath and changed clothes, sitting in a meditative position he told his children and grandchildren that he is leaving for a place called Nether. Then he closed his eyes. A month later he still sat there looking like he was meditating. When people were ready to bury him his body vanished. Only his clothes were left behind.

There are more stories handed down over thousands of years telling a truth that Chinese medicine is a heaven's gift. My desire is to let this profound knowledge benefit all humans on earth. From my own experience of practicing Chinese medicine I deeply feel this knowledge is full of wisdom and power. There is no harsh treatment in Chinese medicine and it is safe and affordable. It won't cost you a fortune to be cured. Chinese medicine works so well in treating chronic diseases and preventing unnecessary surgeries. For all chronic health problems you can find a cure in Chinese medicine.

Doctors and medical insurance cannot guarantee that you won't get sick or be cured. Staying healthy has nothing to do with money or health care condition. Money cannot guarantee that you will suffer less or ensure that you can escape death. Facing a deadly disease no one can say he is rich. One celebrity who could afford the best known experts in the world but she couldn't survive uterine cancer. A rich man with 600 million couldn't buy one inch of healthy intestine and died of colon cancer. Another rich man had two liver transplants that didn't keep him alive. You don't have to be rich to stay healthy. Most healthy and longevity people are hard-working people. Longevity regions in this world are places far from metropolitan areas.

In a longevity village of China, people at old age keep working, eat simple food such as vegetables, bean curd, rice wine, and have never heard about fast food and vitamins. Women never had mammograms done and no one got breast cancer. Nobody suffers osteoporosis or Alzheimer's disease. They have no money, no stress, or anger. They just live a simple, peaceful life.

In this country health care issues perplex most families, and people worry about the money they make is not enough to cover their medical costs. Even for those who can afford vacations at luxurious resorts know the beds in the hospitals are the most expensive beds. Obamacare is also known as affordable health care. It seems with Obamacare more people are able to afford to have health insurance with every month low payment by enroll Obamacare, but when you really need medical attention you may not be able to pay the expensive deductibles. Most discussions regarding of health care are focus on health insurance, in fact the real problem is in this country health insurance only cover one medical system and it is a very expensive medical system. This medical system lack of capacity of cure and the side effects of their drugs make sick people sicker.

In my practice I saw so many people helplessly watching their loved ones suffering illness but they have no idea what they can do to help. Every person should take responsibility for his or her own health. People should have some knowledge about human body and how to take care of themselves. When wild animals get sick they know where to find the herbs to heal themselves, this is the instinct to survive in nature, your pets have already lost their self-healing capacity and they have also lost their ability to access food. Western medicine only has a few hundred years of history. Before modern medicine made available to all people, families relied on women for healing and women took care of sick men and the children with natural remedies. With the development of science and technology, humans are losing their abilities as well. Once sick most people overly rely on doctors and prescription drugs. Many people in the last couple of years of their lives they went through surgeries, consumed a large amount of harmful drugs, suffered a great deal, and spent all of their life savings, leaving their loved ones a large debt and unwillingly died. This is a very sad ending.

Having good health does not mean you have everything, but if you lose your health you could easily lose everything. American people are hard-working people. To make American dreams become reality most people focus their attention on their education, career, business, and gain a long list of material things. If you look at your health as 1, after that 1 you write down a 0 to represent an accomplishment you made in your life, such as your career, your business, owning a house, owning a car, a good marriage, family, … etc., then you could get a big number

1,000,000,000 that is a good fortune. But once you lose that 1 what is left are many zeros. Zero is zero. When you lose your health you could easily lose everything. All those zeros are built on that 1, without that 1 all those zeros just mean zero. Today's reality for most people myself included cannot afford to be sick. A survey shows 60% of bankruptcy filings in the US are due to medical debt. Almost all diseases which doctors say are incurable have cure in this book. If In one family there is one person has the knowledge of food therapy he or she can benefit the whole family. In Chinese medicine food therapy plays an important role in treating diseases and maintaining good health. In this book you can find food remedies to treat almost all health issues at very low cost. Some ingredients can get even be free. With this wonderful book you can free yourself from poor health, prescription drugs, unnecessary surgeries and medical cost.

This book contains some remarkable remedies that have never been taught in medical schools or proven by scientific studies, but they were tested by millions of sick and dying Chinese people who were late stage of cancer patients, kidney failure patients, diabetic patients, and the people who suffered all kinds of illness; in most cases after they spent all of their life savings for their hospital stay and harmful treatments they were sent back home waiting for their final days. Somehow they got these simple remedies that saved their lives and made them healthy again. Some of these remedies were passed down in families from generation to generation as secret treasures, some remedies have been spread among the working people to bring the sick and the dying people back to life and good health. Behind these simple remedies are incredible stories of miracle. I have been collecting natural remedies for years and have shared many remedies with other people in my practice, and also tried some on myself to check their effectiveness.

Nature provides all we need to live on this planet, air, water, food, and medicine. There are abundant herbs that can be used to treat all kinds of human diseases. They are safe, effective, and low cost. They grow in the mountains, by the rivers, or even in our backyards. What we need is to have some knowledge and discover the nature around us. You have free will to decide to rely on your doctors or use your own power to overcome the diseases. For people in serious health condition, they may need doctors to do surgeries or other treatments to save their lives from life threatening stage. This part is only 30% of the whole healing process. The other 70% of the healing process is to gain their strength and regain the normal function of their organic systems which depend on the patients themselves and their loved ones to use food therapy and exercises to win the battle of fighting the diseases. In 2003 my sister got breast cancer and had a surgery. When I went to a cancer hospital in Beijing to visit her I received a lot of information that were passed around by cancer patients and their relatives. The information includes food remedies to enhance the immunity, remedies for replenishing energy and nourishing blood, and the remedy to promote white blood cell growth during and after chemo therapy, etc. We tried some and found they do bring good results.

In all cooking culture there is the knowledge of using food for healing. I would like to use this book to introduce some foods with therapeutic effects that are not well known in western culture. In this book I also use simple language and common sense to explain the diseases and the therapeutic effects of food. You don't need medical background to understand this book, and use it to take care of yourself and help others.

I checked many books about food for healthy living in the market. Those books provided information on which kind of foods contain which kind of nutrients but I noticed the information they are missing is how to prepare the food for healing purposes. Using different way to process food the result can be quite different. Certain foods are used as fresh or dried, or eaten raw or cooked are have different therapeutic effects. Fire is a very powerful energy. Most foods cooked over fire contain more energy than raw food. Frozen foods have lost a lot of their energy. We know lemon rich is in vitamin C also is an alkaline food. Consuming lemon can increase alkaline in our bodies to keep us healthy and prevent cancer. But if drinking a lot of lemon ice tea, like most people do you only get vitamin C unless you drink hot lemon tea that can change the body's PH. In western society people consume more cold and raw food. In China people eat more hot and cooked food. Cold and raw food will cost more energy in the process of metabolism. Energy is invisible to our physical eyes. Homemade meals contain more energy than fast food, because fast foods are processed through mass production in cold metal machines, they can fill up the stomach but they do not provide nourishing and healing energy. Homemade meals are made by people, when they are preparing the meals they put their energy into the food. Fresh grains stored for a long time are losing energy. Frozen food has much less energy than fresh food. The traditional way to prepare the Chinese herbal remedy is to put raw herbs in a pot and cook for about twenty minutes, and then drink the decoction when it is warm. You will see many food remedies are prepared the same way.

Chapter One

Do Vitamins Do More Harm Than Good?

The reason I use the first chapter to talk about vitamins is because today taking vitamins and supplements has become a healthy life style. A lot of people spend more money on vitamins and supplements than they spend on food. In this country people are taught by doctors, TV commercials and online advertising that vitamins and supplements can make them immune to all kinds of diseases. Even healthy people start to take vitamins and supplements at a young age. In this country the production and selling of chemical drugs, vitamins, and supplements is a huge market. Vitamins and supplements are not only sold at drug stores they are also sold at grocery stores and department stores. Some vitamins made in the United States are selling in some drug stores in China as well but with regard to taking vitamins Chinese are not as serious as Americans. Chinese people have the reputation of enjoying cooking and eating everything they can get, those flying in the sky, those swimming in the water, and those running on the land, it is not easy to convince them taking vitamins. American people are very conscious about health, a lot of

Americans spend time working out at gyms, spending more money eating organic food, and taking vitamins. Some studies already raise the question "Do vitamins do more harm than good?" In my practice some people during their first visit show me a long list of vitamins and supplements they have been taking for years. I ask a question to all of them "Since you have been taking these vitamins and supplements for years, do you feel your health is getting better or worse?" All of them have the same answer "My health is getting worse that's why I came to see you." Among all of their health concerns they all have poor digestion and skin problems. On their skin I can see swollen and broken blood vessels, moles, cysts and nodules. According to the theory of Chinese medicine those skin problems are due to the toxic blood. Over consuming vitamins can damage the metabolic system and accumulate toxins in the body. The metabolic system does the work of transforming the food into the nutrients and the work to remove the waste out of the whole body system. If you have some basic knowledge of cell biology you will know removing the waste from the system is a quiet complicated task. Why in this country there is a large population is overweight, even children are out of shape? I believe lack of exercise or unhealthy diet is not the real cause of obesity. Parents with poor metabolism can affect the health of their children and people started taking vitamins from very early age most likely is the cause of damaged metabolism.

16

Do you believe in your doctors or trust your own metabolic systems? Our metabolic systems are very intelligent, they only produce an exact amount of vitamins, protein, and enzymes according to our bodies need and the production is controlled by **negative feedback.** Because the extra products are considered as waste that must be eliminated from our bodies otherwise those unnecessary products remain in the body could cause serious problems, too. For example, we know the pancreas produce insulin. The pancreas does not constantly produce insulin around the clock. It acts by following **negative feedback**. That means only when the amount of insulin in the body is below the normal level the pancreas starts to produce insulin. When the amount of insulin reaches to normal level the pancreas stops to produce insulin, otherwise if the pancreas constantly produces insulin without negative feedback control, insulin level will be higher than the normal and can cause Hypoglycemia which is an abnormal condition as well. So for many diabetic people the fact is daily insulin injections are killing the pancreas. Every day insulin injections make their bodies stored more than enough insulin and their pancreases do not need to produce insulin. For a long period of time their pancreases do not function anymore. This is how people ruined their metabolic systems. Negative feedback also applies to the operation of other organic systems. To treat diabetes the approach of Chinese medicine is to reinforce the function of organic systems.

The history of vitamins dates back to the 1740's. One of the scientists involved in vitamins research was James Lind of Scotland. Lind was a doctor who works for the British Navy. He was trying to solve a problem the Navy had been suffering for hundreds of years. The problem was the disease scurvy. Because many British sailors were suffering scurvy the Navy's fighting strength was very low. The sailors were weak from chronic internal bleeding and their teeth fell out. Even the smallest wound would not heal. Dr. Lind discovered the sailors were getting sick because they were unable to eat some kinds of foods when they were at sea for many months. Through food experiment sailors were cured by eating the fruits which are rich in vitamin C. The study of vitamins continued and the scientists discovered Vitamin A, the B group, C, D, E, K, proteins, enzymes, and also created a huge vitamin market. But today we are living in 21th century and we always have a variety of food supply, so as the sailors. Should we instead of enjoying fresh food but take pills?

Vitamin absorption and utilization should be balanced. Adequate vitamins are very beneficial to general health but long-term or excessive intake of certain vitamins can cause metabolic disorder and lead to disease caused by vitamin imbalance. For example:

1. Vitamin A overdose can cause poisoning. The symptoms include headaches, irritability, nausea, and vomiting. Babies could have cerebral edema,

increased intracranial pressure, fever, sweating, loss of appetite, and skin rash. Every day vitamin A overdose for more than 6 months can cause chronic poisoning symptoms such as pain in the limbs, weight loss, dry hair, losing hair, itchy skin, blurred vision, liver and spleen enlargement, and swelling of the body.

2. Vitamin D overdose can cause headaches, loss of appetite, nausea, vomiting, thirst, polyuria, dehydration, high fever, coma, and urine containing protein and red blood cells. If a pregnant woman overdoses on vitamin A and D can cause the fetus skeletal dysplasia and congenital cataracts. The newborn baby could have hypercalcemia and mental retardation.

3. Vitamin B1 overdose can cause dizziness, edema, diarrhea, and irregular heartbeat. A pregnant woman with an overdose of vitamin B1 can have postpartum bleeding.

4. Vitamin B2 overdose can cause kidney dysfunction.

5. Folate (a vitamin in vitamin B group) overdose can cause bitter taste in the mouth, anxiety, and sleeping disorder.

6. Vitamin B12 overdose can cause asthma, skin rash, chest pain and heart palpitation.

7. Vitamin C long-term overdose can cause nausea, vomiting, abdominal pain, and diarrhea, and suddenly reduce vitamin C intake will be more likely

to cause scurvy. Infant overdose of vitamin C can cause restless sleep, poor digestion, diarrhea, edema, and skin rash.

8. Constant Vitamin E overdose (daily dosage 400mg) could cause thrombus, or lead to menorrhagia or amenorrhea.

Another reason I do not take vitamins is because one of the functions of the metabolic system is to eliminate toxins from the body. Any unwanted substances should be removed. A lot of people think they don't know what kinds of vitamins their bodies need so they taking multivitamins every day. They believe the vitamins which their bodies don't need can eliminate through urination. Among vitamins some substances are water soluble like vitamin C which can be easily get rid of through urination. Some substances are fat soluble and need more complicated processes to eliminate them from the body. Over-consuming vitamins and supplements can cause toxins to accumulate in the body that could lead to cells aging and cancer. Scientific studies discovered in all elderly people's bodies have cancer cells but there are no cancer cells to be found in a new born baby's body. Because a new born baby's blood is so pure that the cancer cells cannot stay alive in an environment without toxins. In the last couple of decades the number of children diagnosed with autism significantly increased. Scientific research has been conducted and found that many toxic chemicals are linked to autism. And autistic children have many dead or poorly functioning brain cells which due to poor protein digestion and toxic overload. How are so many pregnant women and children exposed to toxic chemicals? For all kinds of diseases in most cases the toxins most likely get into the body through the mouth. Sometimes even the most common food and vitamins can become harmful. There is a story circulate on the internet.

In Macao, a girl was dead suddenly and she was bleeding from her eyes, nose, mouth, and ears these are the symptoms of poisoning death. Autopsy report said the cause of death is Arsenic poisoning. After the experts studied the sample taken from the girl's stomach, they identified that this case was not suicide or homicide, but because of ignorance. The Arsenic that killed the girl was produced inside the girl's body. The girl took vitamin C daily. That day she ate a lot of shrimp and took vitamin C at the same time. Shrimp is a very common sea food. Vitamin C is the most common supplement people take. Even many drinks contain vitamin C. Both shrimp and vitamin C are harmless to human body but they can become toxic substances once they combine together.

Shrimp and other soft-shelled sea food contain higher concentration of five potassium arsenic compounds, this substance itself has no toxic effect on the human body but if five potassium arsenic and vitamin C combine together they can produce chemical reaction, non-toxic five potassium arsenic become toxic three potassium arsenic (potassium oxide), that is arsenic. Arsenic can cause paralysis of capillaries, damage liver, causing heart, liver, and kidney blood congestion. Many people say that this story is fictional, I believe so. Because the amount of shrimp and vitamin C the girl consumed would not produce enough Arsenic to cause death, but according to the theory of science it is correct. If eating shelled seafood with vitamin C for a long time could cause chronic poisoning with the symptoms of fatigue, numbness of the limbs, anemia, and kidney dysfunction.

People with normal health condition and keep a balanced diet do not need vitamin supplements. A balanced diet is on the base of a person's physical constitution to eat a small amount of a variety of food. The following are some foods should avoid eating together within two hours.

*Excessive consuming of shrimp with Vitamin C or Vitamin C rich food could lead to chronic poisoning.

*Taking cold medicine with coke could lead to poisoning.

*Long-term eating of chicken eggs with sweetener could lead to poisoning.

*Eating chicken eggs with anti-inflammation medicine could lead to poisoning.

*Eating Tofu (bean curd) with honey can cause deafness.

*Eating peanuts excessively with cucumber can cause damage to kidneys.

*Taking medicine with alcohol can lead to serious consequences.

*Taking cold medicine with alcohol can cause liver failure.

*Taking sleeping pills with alcohol could cause death. Sleeping pills can inhibit breathing and heartbeat. The combination of the two can intensifies inhibition. The patient could have symptoms as slow response, lethargy, decreased blood pressure, respiration slows down, shock, even stop breathing.

*Taking antibiotic medicine with alcohol can lead to poisoning. Five to ten minutes after taking Cephalosporin anti-inflammatory drugs and alcohol, the patient can have symptoms as red complexion, abdominal pain, nausea, decreased blood pressure, shock, and could lead to death. The symptoms can last 30 minutes to several hours.

*Taking lower blood glucose medicine with alcohol can cause low blood glucose and shock. Alcohol can enhance the action of the medicine. Drinking alcohol while taking medication can be life threatening.

*Taking blood pressure medicine with alcohol can cause low blood pressure and shock. Alcohol has the effect of dilating blood vessels and enhancing the effect of anti-hypertension drugs, causing headaches and even shock.

Some lower blood pressure medicine in conjunction with alcohol could cause blood pressure to increase rapidly.

*Taking cardiovascular medicine Nitroglycerin with alcohol can cause low blood pressure and increase blood lipids. Nitroglycerin makes blood vessels expand rapidly. Nitroglycerin used in conjunction with alcohol can cause headaches, decreased blood pressure, elevated blood lipids, gastrointestinal discomfort, and could lead to life threatening situation.

*Some drugs with strong liver toxicity, such as tetracycline, chloramphenicol, erythromycin, anti-TB drugs, anti-neoplastic drugs, and some anti-inflammatory drugs when used in conjunction with alcohol may increase damage to the liver.

*Eating fish or crab with pumpkin can cause food poisoning.

*Eating raw fish with milk can cause food poisoning.

*Eating crab with peanuts or crab with cold food can cause diarrhea.

*Eating crab with sweet potato can cause stones.

*Eating garlic or onion with honey can cause damage to the eyes.

*Eating tomato with sweet potato can cause vomiting, abdominal pain, diarrhea, and stones.

*Eating shrimp with pumpkin can cause Dysentery.

*Taking medicine with milk may affect the efficacy of the drug.

*Eating Tofu or chives with honey can cause diarrhea.

*Drinking milk with acidic drinks (like orange juice) decreases the PH of milk. Acidic drinks cause the protein in milk coagulation that is not conducive to digestion and absorption.

*Drinking milk with chocolate, calcium in milk and the oxalic acid in chocolate combine to generate calcium oxalate that can lead to calcium deficiency and slow growth.

*Drinking milk with spinach can cause Dysentery.

*Always eating meal with soda can cause poor metabolism.

*Drinking alcohol with milk can cause fatty liver and produce toxic substances.

*Drinking alcohol with sugar leads to increased glucose.

*Drinking alcohol with beer can cause stomach cramps, Duodenitis, acute gastroenteritis, and could be very harmful to the cardiovascular system.

*Drinking alcohol with beef could cause internal heat and gum infection.

*Drinking alcohol with carrot could cause hepatotoxicity.

*Drinking beer with seafood can cause Gout.

*Do not drink tea immediately after eating meat. Tea contains a large number of target acid proteins that can cause fatty liver.

The human body can do magic. Its digestive system can transform different food into vitamins, proteins and enzymes according to the body's need. **Be at peace. Let your body does the perfect work!**

Chapter Two

Therapeutic effect of Food

Lamb

I agree that vegetarian food is beneficial to health. I decided to include lamb in this book because its therapeutic effect is better than herbal remedies. Lamb is very beneficial to kidney and stomach. Eating lamb can expel cold from the body, boost energy and replenish blood. Lamb stew is very effective for treating depression and anemia. For symptoms such as lower back pain, weak lower extremities, urination disorders, enlarged prostate and sexual dysfunction, by eating lamb stew all symptoms can be improved in a short period of time.

Lamb Stew Recipe for Depression

In western medicine practice there is no cure for depression, and anti-depressant medication has serious side effects. So far the cause of depression is unknown to western medical study and depression cases are treated as mental illness. In fact depression is due to energy deficiency and triggered by some stressful experiences. A person must have good energy to have a clear mind and be active. Depression is not difficult to be cured. According to

27

my practice records those depression patients who were taking anti-depressant medication for 10 to 20 years all quit anti-depressant medication in one month after received a few treatment sessions, a few bottles of Chinese Herbal remedies, and use this food remedy. If you eat one bowl of lamb stew a day for two weeks you will feel strong enough to stop taking anti-depressant medication. The way of preparing food will affect its therapeutic effect. For therapeutic purpose lamb stew is the best way to eat lamb.

Ingredients: 150 grams lamb cut into small pieces, 10 slices of fresh ginger, ½ cup of black beans

Soak the black beans in cold water overnight. Put lamb, black beans, and the ginger in a pressure cooker. Add water about two inches over the meat. You may add other of your favorite root vegetables, such as carrot, cassava, or potato. Cook over high heat until the water is boiling turn to the low heat cook for 15 minutes. Before eat add some salt for flavor.

You can add other vegetables but lamb and ginger are important ingredients.

Chen Pi (dried tangerine peel)

Chen Pi is dried tangerine peel. Its therapeutic effects are very well known among the Chinese but in the western world they were throw away as waste. When I was very young I already learned tangerine peel is herb. We save them and sell them to the pharmacy. Tangerine peel is thinner than orange peel. I don't know if orange peel has the same therapeutic effects as tangerine peel. I tried orange peel and I noticed Chen Pi has to be made by tangerine peel. Dried tangerine peels are used in some Chinese herbal remedies to treat digestion problems and lung related ailments. I always save tangerine peels and leave them on a paper tower until they completely dry then store them in a glass jar. If someone in my family has stomach discomfort, such as stomach bloating, fullness in the chest, even heart palpitation, I will use Chen Pi to make tea and the symptoms will subside quickly. If your Chen pi has been kept for a long time, for example 2 to 3 years don't throw them away because they have even better healing effects. Chen Pi is like red wine the older the better.

The benefits of Chen Pi include harmonizes stomach, strengthen the function of Spleen, and remove the stagnant gas in digestive system. Symptoms like stomach or abdominal distention, fullness in the chest, bloating, belching, nausea and vomiting are due to stagnant gas in digestive system. This herb promotes the movement of Qi (energy or gas) in general and especially directing the gas downward. Other benefits include drying dampness and transforming phlegm. Treats cough with profuse sputum, stifling sensation in the chest due to lung dysfunction, Loss of appetite, fatigue, and loose stools, cook Chen Pi in boiling water for 15 minutes and drink the hot decoction as tea.

Shan Zha (Hawthorn fruit)

Shan Zha is a fruit that is very well known by Chinese people for its therapeutic effect but it is not recognized in western food culture. The fresh Shan Zha is in deep red color with a strong sweet and sour taste. Like vinegar, lime and lemon, Shan Zha is an alkaline food. In the United States it is hard to find fresh Shan Zha. You can find dried Shan Zha and many snacks made of Shan Zha in Chinese supermarkets. As fruit Shan Zha can be eaten raw or to make healthy and tasty food products or drinks. As an herb to treat ailments we use dried Shan Zha. Having Shan Zha in your diet can promote metabolism, strengthen immunity, and prevent cancer. As an herb its therapeutic function can benefit liver, spleen, and stomach.

Shan Zha can benefit stomach and spleen by eliminating food stagnation due to excessive consuming of meat or greasy food, with symptoms of abdominal distention, belching, poor appetite, and stomachache. It is the best food for weight loss. Charred Shan Zha can be used to treat chronic dysentery-like disorder, and stop diarrhea.

The benefits of Shan Zha for liver include dissipating blood stasis and clots. It is used for eliminating clots and stopping postpartum abdominal pain, or menstrual pain with blood clots due to blood stagnation. As an herb it is also used in certain herbal remedies to treat high blood pressure, high cholesterol, coronary artery disease and fatty liver.

Natural Remedy for Sleep Apnea

Sleep Apnea is a medical term indicating a serious snore problem. People that snore loudly most likely also have other health issues such as poor digestion, obesity, low energy, depression, etc. The real cause of this problem is low energy. In Chinese medicine one diagnosis method is to observe the patient's tongue. If a person's tongue looks swollen with teeth marks along the border that indicates the person's energy is deficient. Without sufficient energy to hold the tissues of the organs the respiratory tract can collapse when the person is relaxed. When the person is sleeping on his back the tongue will drop to the throat to block the airway. The person's sleep partner can notice when this person's energy is better he will snore less, when he is tired he will snore louder. People with hypertension, high cholesterol, obesity, cardiovascular diseases or cough with sputum all can get impressive results by using this remedy. Elderly people having brown spots on their skin that is due to dysfunction of the liver leading to toxins accumulated in the body. Using this remedy can benefit liver and improve skin condition.

The two ingredients of this remedy have the benefits of soothing liver, promoting blood and energy circulation, and eliminating phlegm. This remedy also can improve the condition of shallow breathing and stiffness in the chest. Drinking this decoction regularly can lower blood pressure and LDL cholesterol, promote metabolism, and loss of weight.

Ingredients: 40 grams dried Shan Zha (Hawthorn), 10 grams Chen Pi (dried Tangerine Peel)

Put dried Shan Zha and Chen Pi in a cooking pot, and add 3 cups of water. Cook over high heat until the water is boiling, turn to low heat and cook for 15 minutes. Turn off the heat and pour the decoction in a mug, and add one tea spoon of honey. Drink the decoction when it is warm. It tastes delicious. The same ingredients can be cooked 2-3 times. Minor snoring conditions can be improved on the same day. For serious conditions drink one cup of the decoction in the evening, you will see improvement in a few days.

Fresh Ginger Root

In grocery stores you can find fresh ginger roots in the vegetable section. In Chinese herbal medicine ginger root is used in some herbal remedies as an herb. Ginger root has amazing therapeutic effects but there is a saying that eating ginger in the morning is very good for health, eating ginger in the evening over time could be harmful. The benefits of ginger include:

1. Fresh ginger has the function of detoxification and expels cold. When cooking meat we can add some ginger to avoid food poisoning and get rid of fishy smells. Because ginger is acrid and hot in nature, we can use it to expel cold and harmonize stomach. If after eating cold food such as sea food or certain fruit feel stomach bloating, abdominal pain, diarrhea, or vomiting occurs drink hot ginger tea can help to relieve the symptoms. When you eat at a Japanese sushi restaurant you can always find pickled ginger at sushi bar. The purpose of Japanese restaurants place pickled ginger at the sushi bar is not just for flavor but also for avoiding food poisoning.

   Use ginger to treat diarrhea: There are different types of diarrhea. The diarrhea that is caused by eating the wrong food often accompanied with pain and the cramps in abdomen and the stool with very bad smell. Another type of diarrhea is cold-induced diarrhea that usually happens in the morning due to stomach was exposed to cold air during the night, or after consume too much cold food. This type of diarrhea the stool is very watery without foul smell. In this case drink hot ginger tea can get immediate relief. We can also use ginger to treat common cold, flu, and cough.

   For strengthening energy, promoting circulation and warming up cold limbs: people who suffer cold or numbness of hands and feet can cook fresh ginger in boiling water for five minutes and use the very warm decoction to soak hands and feet, the benefit also include relieving stress and getting better sleep.

2. For losing hair: When you see your hair becoming very thin and falling, you can use a piece of fresh ginger to massage your scalp. Promoting blood circulation of the scalp can stop hair loss.

3. For poor digestion: If you have no appetite and feel stomach bloating after meals. This is due to weakness of the stomach Qi and slow metabolism. By drinking hot ginger tea the condition can improve immediately.

4. Neck pain, shoulder pain, and upper back pain, even toothache very often are caused by stress or poor blood circulation related to heart. Drinking hot ginger tea can dilate blood vessels, promote blood circulation, and reduce the pain.

5. If you have problems, such as cough with white sputum, or watery mucus running out of the nose this is due to cold accumulation in the lungs and lung Qi (energy) deficiency. Drink hot ginger tea can warm up the lung and eliminate the phlegm.

6. For mouth ulcers, gum inflammation, foul smell in the mouth, and sore throat, use hot ginger tea to rinse the mouth 2-3 times per day. Drinking

ginger tea can eliminate inflammation in a few days.

7. For migraine headache and arthritis pain in hands, use hot ginger decoction to soak the hands. You can get relief in 15 minutes. For high blood pressure, use hot ginger decoction to soak the feet 15 minutes in the evening. Do it every day can help balance blood pressure.

8. To get rid of acne on the face, use warm ginger decoction to wash your face in the morning and in the evening for 60 days.

9. To treat Onychomycosis: Onychomycosis is a fungal infection of the nail. Ginger root and vinegar can be used for sterilization. Cook fresh ginger in boiling water for 5 minutes, wait till the water cools down then add some vinegar. Use the decoction to soak the feet.

   By the way rotten ginger contains carcinogens that may induce liver cancer or esophageal cancer.

Dried Chinese Dates (Jujube)

Chinese date is a very popular fruit in China. Chinese people call dried date Da Zao. Da Zao is listed in Chinese herbal medicine books as an herb which is very rich in nutrients. Its therapeutic effects are very well known by Chinese people, especially Chinese women are taught that Da Zao nourishes blood and they should have dates in their everyday diet for good health and to keep a youthful appearance. In summer at the dates harvest season Chinese people eat fresh dates, the rest of the year they eat dried dates. Fresh dates and dried dates have different therapeutic effects. Dried dates contain more nutrients than fresh dates. Dried dates contain vitamin A, B2, C, Calcium, phosphorous, and iron. In the United States you can find dried dates in Chinese supermarkets. Dried dates can strengthen the function of spleen. According to the theory of Chinese medicine the function of spleen is to transform food to energy and blood. Spleen deficiency will cause the symptoms like anemia, low energy, short of breath, lassitude, poor appetite, and loose stools. In some Chinese herbal remedies dried dates are used for nourishing blood and calming the mind to treat restlessness, irritability, and unbalanced emotions. Da Zao also plays a role in some herbal remedies to protect spleen and stomach, and to eliminate side effects from other herbs.

According to the theory of Chinese medicine, Hepatitis and Cirrhosis are caused by poor nutrition and liver blood deficiency. A clinic records show patients with high serum transaminase levels from either Hepatitis or Cirrhosis were given dried Chinese dates and peanuts decoction with brown sugar for a month. By the end of that time the transaminase level were significantly decreased in all the patients. Over the last a couple of decades, dried Chinese dates become a very important ingredient in food therapy for cancer patients.

Da Zao is a very nutritious food that should be kept in a refrigerator to avoid infestation.

Gou Qi Berry (Wolfberry)

Gou Qi berries are small red berries. Dried Gou Qi berries look like raisins and taste sweet. Like blueberry and raspberry, Gou Qi berry is fruit but in Chinese herbal medicine it is listed as one of the top grade herbs because of its therapeutic effects and without any side effects. It has played an important role in some very common used herbal remedies and food remedies. It is very well known by Chinese people because of its anti-aging effect especially those people who are over age 40, many of them keep Gou Qi berry in their diet to maintain good health and youthful appearance. In Chinese history there is a record of the most long-lived man who lived 256 years on earth. His name was Qing Yun Li (1677-1933). His photos which are kept in the archives of the local government show he was nine feet tall and burly. In his long life he had 24 wives and 180 children and grandchildren. At age 10 he started traveling to different states collecting herbs. He specialized in treating eye diseases and orthopedics. He practiced Chinese medicine and sold herbs to make a living. Later he became a Chinese medicine scholar. In 1777 at age 100 he obtained a special award from the government because of his outstanding achievement in Chinese medicine. At age 200 he still gave lectures at the university and accepted western scholars' visits. He was kind and never got angry. How can he live such a long life? He said the first reason for his longevity is he is a vegetarian. The second reason is he always maintains a peaceful mind. The third reason is he drinks the Gou Qi berry decoction every day.

Gou Qi berry contains more than 18 amino acids and carotenes that are main components in making antibodies, hormone, and blood cell formation. Gou Qi berries are very beneficial to liver and kidney. Gou Qi berry promotes the function of liver, lower LDL cholesterol to prevent arteriosclerosis. People with diabetes add Gou Qi berries in every day diet can balance blood glucose. According to the theory of Chinese medicine all symptoms of aging are related to the kidney essence deficiency. The symptoms like pain in lower back and legs, the weak knees, osteoporosis, gray hair and losing hair, losing memory, slow metabolism, blurred vision and diminished visual acuity, tinnitus (ringing in the ear), sexual dysfunction, frequent urination or difficult urination, plus aging linked diseases, such as hypertension and diabetes, etc. Gou Qi berry is a super food for replenishing the essence of the liver and the kidney. By adding Gou Qi berry in daily diet all symptoms can be improved in a short period of the time. For elderly people having Gou Qi berry in their diet can brighten the eyes, strengthen the bones and the ligaments, and slow down the aging process. As an herb Gou Qi berry doesn't have any side effects and it has been used in many Chinese herbal remedies. Over the last couple of decades, in the battle of fighting cancers Chinese medical records show Gou Qi berry has the power to inhibit cancer cell growth and protect white blood cells. Today in China Gou Qi berry has become one of the most important herbs being used in food therapy to help cancer patients to enhance their immunity and reduce the side effects of chemotherapy.

Remedy for Varicose Veins

Varicose veins are commonly developed in legs. Some prescription drugs can cause damage to veins. Laser treatment and compression stockings do not treat its underlying cause.

Soak 50 grams of Gou Qi berries in a bottle of alcohol for two weeks. Every day apply the remedy on affected area with 5 minutes light massage. Varicose veins can completely disappear in 3 to 6 months.

Black Sesame Seed

Black sesame seed is not popular in western cooking culture but in China It is a favorite food for Chinese people because of its therapeutic and anti-aging effects. Both black and white sesame seeds have therapeutic effects for maintaining good health but according to Chinese medicine theory foods with black color like black sesame seed, black rice and black beans are especially beneficial to kidney and have more anti-aging effect than other colored food. Black sesame seeds are powerful antioxidant food and rich in vitamin E. Having black sesame seeds in your diet also can protect your heart. Unsaturated fatty acids and Lecithin in black sesame seed helps maintaining elasticity of blood vessels and prevent arteriosclerosis. It has great benefits for liver and kidney as well. All aging related symptoms such as gray hair or losing hair, blurred vision, tinnitus, osteoporosis, losing memory, etc. are due to deficiency of the kidney essence and black sesame seed can replenish kidney essence. Black sesame seed contains iron and variety of vitamins that nourish blood to benefit liver and kidney. Black sesame seed also has therapeutic effect of strengthening muscles, bones and tendons. Another benefit of black sesame seed is moistening and lubricating the intestines to relief constipation caused by blood deficiency or the dryness of the intestines. Over all black sesame seeds are super food that enhance immunity and prevent aging. Add this food in the diet of the aged and frail can help them recover from illness and stay strong.

Black sesame seed is so good for your health but it is difficult for the stomach to digest. If you eat the whole seeds they will go through the body undigested. The best way to get the benefits of the black sesame seed is to eat black sesame seed in the form of powder. When you cook oatmeal (or cornmeal) adding one tablespoon of black sesame powder can make your oatmeal taste better.

Garlic

In Chinese herbal medicine books garlic is listed as a powerful anti-virus herb. It kills intestinal parasites like hookworms and pinworms. Detoxification action of the garlic can stop diarrhea, dysentery, and food poisoning from shellfish. Garlic can be used to treat seafood allergy, asthma, cough with white mucus, and difficult breathing.

Garlic has a very strong antibiotic effect against many pathogenic bacteria. It can effectively kill the bacteria that are resistant to penicillin. Other benefits of Garlic are expelling cold, clearing phlegm, and stopping cough. It is very commonly used in a home remedy to treat common cold and flu among Chinese people. Garlic also has therapeutic effect in treating cardiovascular diseases. Garlic oil inhibits the development of atherosclerosis. Garlic's antifungal effect can bring significant results in treating pathogenic fungi.

Potato

Potato probably is the most common food but most people may not realize potato has magic powers to cure many ailments. Potato is not listed in any herbal medicine book as an herb, but it does have incredible healing power. Potato has the benefits of harmonizing digestive system, boosting energy, and strengthening the function of the kidney. Raw potato can be used to relieve pain, minimize inflammation and swelling of the skin. For Goiter, scar tissue, and shingles, simply cut potato into thin slices and paste them on the neck, scar tissue or the shingles. Potato also can be used to treat gastric ulcer, stomach cancer, and esophageal cancer.

Remedy for Esophageal Cancer

To treat esophageal cancer, peel a medium sized raw potato and cut into small pieces. Put the potato in a blender and add some water just to cover the potato to make potato paste. For esophageal cancer let the patient take one tablespoon of potato paste and hold the potato paste in the mouth, lies down on the back then slowly little by little swallow down the potato paste. Let the potato paste slowly flow down the throat and the esophagus. Use this remedy three times a day to relief pain, diminish inflammation, and swollen.

For people with stomach ulcer and stomach cancer drink one cup of raw potato paste before the meal on empty stomach three times a day, the condition should improve in 1 to 2 weeks. Continue to use this remedy until the ulcer completely heals. For cancer patients drinking raw potato paste has the benefit of strengthening the immune system and inhibiting cancer cell growth. Cancer patients also need use other food therapy to enhance the physical constitution.

For people with severe liver disease or kidney disease drink 1 to 2 cups of raw potato juice per day. The condition can improve quickly. Proteinuria can completely disappear in a couple of days.

Another therapeutic way to use potato is relieve the swelling and pain of the joints. Use a piece of fresh ginger root and one potato together to make the paste. The amount depends on how much you really need. Apply the ginger potato paste on the painful joint and use gauze to wrap the joint at least for half hour. Use this treatment 1 to 2 times a day until the symptoms completely gone.

For other conditions such as scalding, injured muscles, or strained tendons and ligaments all can use raw potato to treat inflammation, swellings and relieve the pain.

Raw potato also can be used to treat skin disorders. For acne apply raw potato paste on affected area to help reduce redness and inflammation. Shingles can be very painful. If you get a shingles outbreak use raw potato paste or cut thin slices of raw potato cover the shingles can help relieve the pain immediately. If you can find a Chinese medicine practitioner make an appointment. In Chinese medicine there are treatment and herbal remedies available for this skin disorder.

Remedy for Kidney Stones

The symptom of kidney stone is pain that starts suddenly when a kidney stone is passing through the urinary tract. This can cause sharp pain or cramping pain in the lower back and the lower abdomen. The cause of kidney stones still remains unknown for conventional medical studies and there is no reliable treatment available for this disease. The doctors' recommendation for the patients with kidney stones is drinking a lot of water which doesn't help to improve the kidney's condition. At one of my "Food as Medicine" lectures a lovely lady shared this remedy with us. This remedy is used by people in South America to treat kidney stones. She got this remedy and used it removed all of her kidney stones.

When we make potato salad or mash potatoes, we peel the potatoes and cook them in boiling water until the potatoes are cooked. Then we remove the potatoes from the water to make potato salad or mashed potatoes. What are you going to do with the water that was used to cook the potatoes? That water is the best medicine to treat kidney stones. By drinking that water kidney stones will melt like sand and be easily released from the body when the patient is urinating.

For people without kidney stones can use that water to make vegetable soup to keep their kidneys strong and healthy. I keep telling people if we look at a human being as a tree, the kidneys are the roots. If the roots of a tree die the tree will die. If a person's kidneys die the person will die. That is why many diseases at the late stage are kidney failure. If you want to live an active long life you must take good care of your kidneys.

Black Bean

Black bean is a very popular food in many cultures. In some ancient Chinese pharmacopoeia black beans have been documented as a food for maintaining youth and beauty. Black beans contain Anthocyanins, a very good source of antioxidants that can eliminate free radicals in the body to slow down aging process. Generally speaking, foods with dark red color or with color black contain Anthocyanins, such as black rice, black sesame seeds, dark red beans, and grapes. Also black beans contain plenty of proteins, vitamin E, vitamin B group, calcium, iron, and lecithin. The benefits of having black beans in your diet includes strengthening the function of kidneys, Lower LDL cholesterol, balance blood pressure, promote blood circulation, softening the blood vessels, regulating blood glucose, preventing hair loss and gray hair, losing memory, blurring vision, tinnitus, and losing hearing.

Black beans also contain Isoflavones that is equivalent to natural female estrogen. Most women around age 50 experience some symptoms of menopausal syndrome due to lack of estrogen. Symptoms include irritability, hot flashes, tiredness, and osteoporosis, etc. Eating more black beans and soybeans can be very helpful at menopausal time.

Caution: Do not eat black beans with milk and spinach. It could cause side effects. People with Gout should avoid black beans in their diet because black beans contain high level of Princeton.

Chi Xiao Dou (Chinese red beans)

Chi Xiao Dou, English translation is dark red little bean. Chinese people call it red bean. Chi Xiao Dou like other beans is food. Because of its therapeutic benefits it is listed in Chinese herbal medicine books as an herb. Chi Xiao Dou is smaller and its red color is darker than the red beans that are sold in supermarkets. So far Chi Xiao Dou can only be found at Chinese supermarkets. According to Chinese herbal medicine Chi Xiao Dou has therapeutic effects on heart and small intestine. Its therapeutic actions include clear heat, promoting urination, balancing blood pressure, detoxification, lowering LDL cholesterol, and regulating blood glucose. It is very beneficial to patients with heart disease, kidney disease, and edema. It can be used to improve the symptoms such as abdominal fullness, difficult urination, and edema in the lower extremities that is due to kidney deficiency. Chi Xiao Dou is also known to contain iron, calcium, and vitamin B complex that is essential for metabolic energy production. Chi Xiao Dou is rich in dietary fiber that helps to moisten the intestine and promote bowel movement. Chi Xiao Dou has a long history of being used as a food remedy for weight loss.

Honey

Honey is a very stable substance, if properly preserved it can keep its quality for hundreds of years without degeneration and its nutrition will not be lost. Honey is the only non-man made sweetener, it has the simplest molecular structure that cannot be further decomposed. From the small intestine it can directly enter the blood so that it won't cause any digestive system disorder. Therapeutic effects of honey are beneficial to lung, heart, liver, spleen, and kidney. It contains amino acids that can reduce fat accumulation in the cardiovascular system to prevent hardening of arteries. Scientific study discovered honey contains several antioxidants and one of them has the anti-aging effect that can only be found in honey. Honey can improve sexual dysfunction which is due to old age or infirmity. Honey can be used to treat burns, relieve pain, and make quick recovery on the affected skin without leaving scars. It is the best natural ingredient for cleansing the skin. Apply some honey evenly on the whole face and leave it there for 10 minutes, then use water to wash it away, the result is like having a facial treatment. The following are some remedies for improving serious health conditions.

1. Squeeze one cup of celery juice, add one teaspoon of honey and stir. Take three times a day, take 1/3 of the juice before the meal to improve the condition of urinary tract stones, prostate disease, and dermatitis.

2. Add one teaspoon of honey in one cup of raw tomato juice and stir. Drink the juice 2 to 3 times per day to promote metabolism, to prevent Atherosclerosis, enhance hematopoietic function, and maintain body acid-base balance.

3. Add one teaspoon of honey in one cup of raw pumpkin juice and stir. Drink 2 to 3 times per day to promote urination to help treating cardiovascular disease, obesity, liver disease, kidney disease, and prostate cancer.

4. One of the commonly seen problems in elderly people is constipation. Add one teaspoon of honey in one cup of raw cucumber juice and drink two to three cups per day to moisten intestines, to promote urination and bowel movement. Long-term use of this remedy can prevent hair loss and Hyperthyroidism which related to aging.

5. People with weak immunity can add one teaspoon of honey in milk to relieve fatigue and enhance immunity. For cancer patients after surgery and during chemo therapy use American ginseng to make tea and add one teaspoon of honey to it, to boost energy and eliminate side effects of chemo therapy.

6. Honey has a therapeutic effect of inhibiting of excessive gastric acid secretion and prevent gastric and duodenal ulcer. In the evening before going to bed drink one small cup of raw potato juice mixed with one teaspoon of honey to promote metabolism and the function of heart, avoid stomach bloating and acid reflux.

Dandelion

Dandelion grows everywhere. People treat dandelion as a weed. In Chinese herbal medicine dandelion is used as an herb. Clinical records show it is beneficial to liver and gallbladder, and has therapeutic effects in treating gallbladder stones and edema. In spring time when I do my morning jogging I will sometimes collect some dandelion to make dumplings or salad. Living in today's fast-paced environment many people complain about the discomfort which is caused by stress, such as irritability, anxiety, poor sleep, and over thinking. According to Chinese medicine theory a person living under a prolonged stress could have toxic heat accumulate in the liver that can lead to the symptoms of irritability, dry mouth and bitter taste in the mouth, poor sleep, and constipation. Eating dandelion salad can clear the toxic heat in the liver and make us more relaxed. Dandelion also can clear the toxic heat in lung to release sore throat as well. Another therapeutic function of dandelion is to treat difficult urination and the burning sensation during urination that is caused by urinary tract infection. Soak dandelion in boiling water for a couple of minutes, drain the water. Add crushed fresh garlic, a little salt and vinegar. Eat as vegetable.

Dandelion also can be used to treat breast abscess. Collect some fresh dandelion and wash them clean. Chop the dandelion or put dandelion in a blender and blend them to paste. Apply the paste on the breast to stop the pain immediately and the breast abscess can be cured in a couple of days.

Mung Beans (Chinese green beans)

Mung beans are very small beans in dark green color. You can only find Mung beans in Chinese supermarkets and Chinese people call them green beans. As an herb the therapeutic effect of Mung beans includes clear summer heat, fever, irritability, and release toxic heat from the body. Cook Mung beans in boiling water for 15 minutes and drink the decoction. The beans are edible.

After my son finished high school he got his first job working at a Dunkin Donuts store. One summer day the air conditioning in the store broke down. Inside of the store was so hot. After work my son came home complaining of headache and nausea. When I find out what happened at his work, I immediately made the Mung beans decoction for him. As soon as he drank the decoction the symptoms were gone.

If you get flu with fever, use Mung beans decoction to reduce the fever. For women who are going through menopause drink Mung bean's decoction to relieve hot flashes. Stress also can cause toxic heat in the body. The symptoms include anxiety, irritability, constipation, dry mouth, and bitter taste in the mouth, by drinking Mung bean's decoction can clear toxic heat and release stress related symptoms.

Vinegar

Vinegar has a long history in Chinese herbal medicinal use. In this book you shall find vinegar appears in many remedies as an important ingredient. Vinegar is an alkaline food that can keep us healthy and slow down the aging process. According to the theory of Chinese medicine the foods with sour taste are beneficial to liver and vinegar is one of them. Adding vinegar in the daily diet helps improve some health problems related to an unhealthy liver. For example, people with Cirrhosis or having cramps in four extremities, blurred vision, high blood pressure, high cholesterol, brown spots on the skin, etc. For maintaining good health eat vinegar often can soften veins to prevent heart disease and stroke.

Osteoporosis is an aging related disease. It affects 1 in 2 women after age 50. Taking calcium and vitamin D supplements sound like make sense in the theory but in a matter of fact it does not really make patient's bone stronger. The bone formation is much more complicated than calcium plus vitamin D. Use ribs to make soup and when cooking ribs add some vinegar in it to make calcium, phosphorus, iron, and other minerals dissolve from the ribs. Cook the soup this way allowing the body to absorb the nutrition easily. Exercise is also very important for people with Osteoporosis.

Pumpkin and Pumpkin Seed

Pumpkin has low calorie and rich in fiber, it is a super food for weight loss. Pumpkin contains carotene which will be transferred to vitamin A in our bodies, and vitamin A is an essential element for Retinol. Pumpkin also contains important material for constituting eye lens. Prolonged use of computer may cause eye fatigue, eating pumpkin has benefits for eyes and prevent cataract. Elderly people have pumpkin in their diet can prevent vision loss. Scientific study discovered that pumpkin is a powerful antioxidant and anti-aging food. It contains plenty of vitamin B1, B2, B6, vitamin C and iron. Add pumpkin in your diet has the benefits of strengthening immunity, balancing blood glucose, and prevent cancer. Oncology research discovered that carotene can reduce the risk of prostate cancer.

Pumpkin seed is a source of unsaturated fatty acids. Eat pumpkin seeds can help to prevent cardiovascular diseases. For women eating pumpkin seeds can promote postpartum fluid metabolism to release postpartum symptoms of swelling hands and feet, and it also can be used to treat insufficient lactation.

Another benefit of pumpkin seeds is expel parasites and alleviates abdominal pain. Add pumpkin seeds in pet's food can expel tapeworms and other intestinal parasites in animals.

Chive and Chive Seed

Chive is also called Chinese leek. Chive has 3000 years of planting history in China. It is an ingredient with strong flavor. Both chive and its seeds are listed in Chinese herbal medicine books as herbs. They are very beneficial to liver and the kidney.

To benefit liver, chive is a blood mover. It can promote blood circulation, lower bad cholesterol, and strengthen immunity. Chive contains flavonoids that make it having bactericidal and anti-inflammatory effects.

To benefit kidney, chive can strengthen the function of the kidney and replenish the essence of the kidney. Add chive in your diet helps to improve the condition of frequent urination and urgent urination. It also helps improving the conditions like sore lower back and weak knees. The seeds of chive have stronger therapeutic effects than the plant. Chive seeds are used in certain Chinese herbal remedies to warm up kidneys, improve functions of the kidneys, replenish kidney essence to treat impotence, spermatorrhea, urinary incontinence, kidney stones, vaginal discharge, and the weakness of lower back and the knees. Seeds can be grounded to powder, take twice a day, each time take 9 grams of the powder to treat impotence and seminal emission. Or cook 15 grams of chive seed powder in boiling water for 10 minutes, and drink the decoction as hot tea.

One of the kidney deficiency symptoms is cold feet. People have kidney stones their feet are cold that indicates the kidney's energy is very low unable to warm up the feet. You don't need go to see your doctor for diagnosis because the tests may show there is nothing wrong with your kidneys. The tests performed in western medicine cannot check the kidney's energy and the kidney's essence level. If western medicine tests show you have kidney disease your kidney is already seriously damaged. Even you do have kidney disease that still can be treated with Chinese medicine and food therapy. After you taking Chinese herbal remedy or drinking the chive seeds decoction your feet will get warm that indicates the condition of your kidneys are improved.

Chive Porridge for Impotence

The function of sexual organs depends on the health of kidney. The cause of Impotence is due to the dysfunction of the kidneys. Taking Viagra can cause more damage to the kidneys. Chive is natural "Viagra". Eating this porridge often can strengthen the energy and improve the function of the kidneys.

Mix 10 grams of chive seeds powder with 100 grams of sticky rice in a cooking pot and add 4 to 5 cups of water. Cook over high heat until the water is boiling, change to the low heat cook until the rice is well cooked. After turn off the heat add a little salt for flavor. If you cannot find chive seeds you may use chives. Take 50 grams of fresh chives chopped and set aside. Cook 100 grams of sticky rice in five cups of water to make porridge first. When the porridge is done turn off the heat then add in chopped chives and a little salt, it is ready for eat.

Remedy for Prolapsed Uterine

Prolapsed uterine refers to the descent of the uterus into the vagina, in some cases the uterus could drop out of the body. This problem due to kidney energy is very deficient or weak constitution lead to a condition that the energy cannot hold the uterus in position. Women with prolapsed uterus must avoid excessive exercise and weight lifting that can make the condition worse. In Chinese medicine there are treatment and herbal remedies available to strengthen energy and lift the uterus up back to the place. During the treatment use food therapy eat well and resting well is important.

This is a remedy for external use. Cook 250 grams of fresh chives in half gallon of boiling water for 10 minutes. Use the warm decoction wash vagina.

The following recipe also can be used to reinforce energy. This is a very commonly used recipe in Chinese cooking culture. It is scramble eggs plus one ingredient Chive. Eat this dish often can strengthen the energy and nourish the blood, it also beneficial to the kidneys and strengthen the weakness of lower back and the knees.

Chive Scramble Eggs Recipe

Scramble eggs is the most common dish for breakfast. Probably you know how to cook perfect scramble eggs, you can use your own way of cooking and add chive in the eggs to increase the therapeutic effect. 100 grams of fresh chives washed and chopped mix with 3 eggs in a bowl stir well, add a little salt. Put 2 table spoons of oil in a pan when the oil is hot pour the eggs into the pan and cook over medium heat for a few minutes, it is done for breakfast.

Remedy for Athlete's Foot

Cut 250 grams of chives one inch long and place the chives in half gallon of the boiling water cook for 5 minutes. Use the chive decoction soaking the feet for 20 minutes a day for three days. The Athlete's foot can be cured.

Remedy for Treating Skin disorders

This remedy is used to treat Hives, Eczema, or itchy skin. When cooking rice save the water that had been used for washing the rice. Place 50 grams of chives in that water and cook for 10 minutes. Use a cotton ball soak the decoction and apply it on the affected skin as many times as you can. You may see the improvement on the same day. Make new decoction every day and keep using the remedy for 7 to 10 days for complete cure.

Water

70% of our planet is made of water so as a human body. Water is so important for life. Water plays an irreplaceable role in the body metabolism. All food we ate must combine with water molecules to transform to the nutrients for body to absorb even waste substances must combine with water molecules to be eliminated from the body. In my practice I noticed many health issues are caused by the wrong way of using water.

First we cannot use beverages to replace water. Many people think there are no nutrients in the pure water. On every kind of beverage bottle there is a label listed the vitamins that are contained in the beverage. Those labels make people to believe fruit juice is more nutritious than water. For their health concern they drink a variety of juices instead of water. Use fruit juice replace water can lead to poor metabolism and other health issues. For women excessive and long-term consumption of carbonated drinks can lead to Osteoporosis. Carbonated beverages can hinder the body's absorption of calcium and lead to the decrease of bone density. If you are old enough you should remember several decades ago, before fruit juices and soda made available everywhere what people drink was water and at that time people were in better shape and healthier.

Here is a real case from my work. A 63-year-old woman at her first visit her complain was irregular bowel syndrome, and had diarrhea every morning. She looked much older than her age. She was overweight with whole body water retention. She always suffering lower back pain and had very bad knees. Her skin was so bad especially her legs with many broken vines, and she was diagnosed having Leukemia. A person's skin reflects the condition of her blood, all skin problems related to poor quality of the blood. She is very serious about her health and tried to avoid taking prescription drugs but she took many different kinds of vitamins and supplements. She also likes to go to health seminars and tried to eat healthy. She spent a lot of money shopping at Whole Food Stores for organic food but she is not good at cooking. Her breakfast was fruit juice and smoothies. I tried convincing her instead of drinking fruit juice and smoothies, drink hot tea or water and eat regular food like oatmeal, egg, and multigrain bread for breakfast. She had hesitated for a few weeks and finally she tried. The first day she had oatmeal and an egg for breakfast she didn't have diarrhea that morning. My advice for her is "don't spoil yourself just eat simple food that provide enough nutrients for your body's need and let your body does the perfect work!"

In eastern culture people prefer to drink hot water and at the old time before refrigerator was invented, people used to drink room temperature water or hot tea, and at that time people were healthier than the population today. Ice cold drink can weaken the function of stomach and spleen. If you have a glass of cold water or cold drink before the meal, the cold temperature makes your stomach contract that will consume stomach energy to warm up before digest the food. That meal will take longer time to digest and can cause acid reflux. If you drink hot tea or hot soup before the meal, your stomach is relaxed and ready to digest food. Only by changing the habit of drinking cold water can avoid stomach bloating and acid reflux. Stomach and spleen are two major organs in metabolic system. Spleen is responsible for transforming food to energy and blood. People who are overweight, have low energy, and upper body retaining water are due to the dysfunction of stomach and spleen. According to the theory of Chinese medicine when stomach Qi (energy) exhausted will lead to sudden death. Many sudden death cases are diagnosed by western medicine as heart attack. In China doctors in both western and eastern medicine have the records that show among those sudden death cases many people had drunk cold drinks such as cold beer, or ate cold water melon before they die. The true cause of their sudden death is not heart attack but the stomach Qi used up. Elderly people must change the habit of drinking cold water. Drinking hot water to protect stomach Qi sounds not a big deal but it does affect life and death.

Should we drink eight glasses of water per day? Many people drink eight glasses water per day because their doctors told them to do so. I think they should listen to their bodies. Swelling of legs and feet are the symptoms of kidney deficiency. When I tell People those symptoms are due to kidney deficiency they would say they will drink more water. If a person's kidneys are deficient and he intentionally drinking a lot of water that only adds more stress on the kidneys. Many people think by drinking more water can solve all health problems unfortunately it is not that simple unless you drink real holy water. The following are some therapeutic ways to use water.

*To prevent acid reflux and stomach bloating drink hot water or hot tea before and after the meal.

*For Migraine headache, soak both hands in hot water and let the water cover the wrists. Headache can be reduced in half an hour.

*For heart palpitation, drink hot water can get relief.

* Ice is another form of water. Many people use ice for pain relief. For most cases this is a wrong therapy especially when used on elderly people. Only treat injury caused the pain with red, hot, and swollen you use ice to relieve the pain and stop swelling. In addition to the pain caused by trauma, most pain is due to poor circulation. Warm temperature can promote blood circulation to relieve pain. Cold temperature will slow down blood circulation that could cause more pain so that the only condition to use ice therapy is to treat injury with swollen.

Lime and Lemon

Lime and lemon are powerful detoxification food. They have strong sour taste and in metabolic system they can make the body constitution slightly alkaline. Lemon and lime are already well known as anti-aging food. They are a good source of vitamin C. Vitamin C helps to eliminate toxins from skin to reduce dark spots on the skin and improve skin condition. Apply a little lemon juice on the nails can make nails strong and shinning. Lemon juice can stop gum bleeding and reduce tooth decay. Drink hot lemon tea can detoxify the liver, prevent gallbladder stones, reduce stress, and promote metabolism to lose weight. Lemon contains potassium that helps balance blood pressure and lower LDL cholesterol. Drink hot lemon tea can strengthen immunity. It is very beneficial to cancer patients.

Hot Lemon Tea Kills Cancer Cells

Ice cold lemonade is a very popular drink. Hot lemon tea sounds not appealing to most of people, but from ice cold lemonade your body only get vitamin C. Hot lemon tea is alkaline water that releases a substance that inhibit the growth of cancer cells. Hot lemon tea also has the benefits of moistening the lungs and ease asthma.

To make hot lemon tea take two lemons washed clean and thinly sliced, place them in a glass jar, add honey and a little cold drinking water to cover the lemon. Seal the jar and store it in a refrigerator overnight. The next day take 2 slices of lemon put them in a cup and pour hot water into the cup to make hot lemon tea.

Soybean

Soybean is one of the essential foods in Chinese people's diet. In China all restaurants that sell breakfast provide a variety of soybean products, such as fresh made soybean milk and soybean curd. Soybeans contain a large number of protein, calcium, fiber, carotene, iron, and phosphorus. It has therapeutic effect of lowering LDL cholesterol in blood. It is very beneficial to the people with coronary heart disease or Arteriosclerosis (hardening of blood vessels).

For children drink soybean milk can promote physical and mental development. For elderly people soybean milk is easier to digest than cow milk. One of the Chinese people's favorite soybean products is fermented bean curd that contains a lot of vitamin B12. As an anti-aging food, it can slow down brain aging and prevent Alzheimer's disease. Soybean milk contains a lot of natural Estrogen that is very beneficial to the women with menopausal syndrome and helps to prevent osteoporosis.

Even soybean dreg can be used to make delicious bread and pan cakes. Soybean dreg contains an anti-cancer substance called Isoflavones that can prevent breast cancer, pancreatic cancer, prostate cancer, and colon cancer.

Soybean Pancake

You can shop online buy a soymilk maker, with a soymilk maker you can easily make fresh soymilk for your breakfast. Each time you make soymilk you will get some soybean dreg. If you have a bread maker you can add soybean dreg with other ingredients to make multigrain bread. If you don't have a bread maker you can make nutritious soybean pancakes.

Ingredients: soybean dreg, 2 tablespoons of flour, 2 eggs, 3 chopped green onions, a little salt

Mix well all ingredients together add a little water to make the paste, the rest you already know how to make pancakes.

Job's tears Seed

Job's tears seed looks like rice with bland taste. It is grain and it is listed in Chinese herbal medicine book as an herb as well. Its therapeutic effects benefit the organs include Spleen, Lung, and Kidney. It is used in some Chinese herbal remedies to treat the symptoms of poor digestion, frequent bowel movement with loose stool and undigested food, lack of energy, and obesity. Having Job's tears seeds in your diet can strengthen the function of the spleen, promote metabolism, promote urination and leach out dampness. Pregnant women should avoid to eat Job's tears seeds because they can cause uterus contraction and lead to miscarriage.

Red Beans and Seed of Job's tears Decoction

Both red beans and Job's tears seeds have the function of promote urination and treat edema. One symptom of Gout is inflammation of the joints that caused by accumulation of uric acid in the body. Job's tears seeds can eliminate the uric acid from the body therefore this remedy can treat Gout and urination disorder. Job's tears seeds also can clear damp-heat in the body to relieve painful obstruction like Rheumatoid arthritis, reduce the swollen of the joints and increase the joints mobility. Clinical research showed Job's tears seed has relaxing effect on striated muscles.

In clinic an often seen case is women complaining of scanty, dark urine with burning sensation. This is caused by damp-heat obstructing urinary bladder channels. Use this remedy to treat this problem is very effective.

This remedy also can be used to treat acne. The cause of acne is related to poor digestion and damp-heat accumulation in the body. Job's tears seeds have the therapeutic effect of strengthening the function of spleen to promote metabolism and promote urination to clear damp-heat.

Another benefit of Job's tears seed is to clear the heat in lungs and expel pus to treat soft pus related carbuncles as well as lung and intestinal abscess. Clinical research showed that Job's tears seed has inhibitory effect on the growth of the cancer cells.

Chinese women use this remedy for weight loss. People who are overweight believe they have extra fat stored in their bodies, in fact in most cases those extra weight are caused by water retention. The good news is to get rid of the water is much easier than get rid of the fat. Keep using this remedy for 1 to 2 weeks your body will be lighter.

Ingredients: 1/3 cup of Chi Xiao Dou (Chinese red beans), 1/3 cup of Job's tears seeds

Soaking Job's tears seeds and Chinese red beans in cold water for two hours. Together put them in a cooking pot and add 5cups of water cooking over high heat until the water is boiling turn to the low heat continue to cook for

30 minutes. Drink the decoction and eat the ingredients. Use this remedy once a day for a few days the condition will improve significantly.

Anti-aging Tea

One cup of Job's tears seeds washed and put in a saucepan bake them over low heat until they turned to light brown. After the baked Job's tears seeds are cool down store them in a container. Each time take 15 grams of baked Job's tears seeds and 10 grams of Gou Qi berries together put in a mug, add in boiling water soaking for 5 to 10 minutes. Drinking this tea often can keep a younger looking.

Longan

Longan is a tropical fruit. It tastes very sweet and rich in nutrients. Dried Longan has stronger therapeutic effect than fresh fruit. Dried Longan is available at Chinese supermarkets. In Chinese herbal medicine Longan is a tonify herb. As an herb it benefits heart and spleen. It is used in food remedies and Chinese herbal remedies for nourishing blood and calm the spirit to treat insomnia, heart palpitation, forgetfulness, and dizziness which is due to heart and spleen deficiency. It is commonly used to treat problems associated with aging and weak constitution. Longan is very a nutritious food which should be stored in a refrigerator to prevent infestation.

Raisin

Laboratory studies showed that grapes can lower blood pressure, strengthen the functions of heart, and eliminate the inflammation in body. Raisin is one of the popular and delicious foods. Add raisin in everyday diet is very beneficial to general health. Raisin nourishes blood to improve the condition of Anemia, constipation, and fatigue. During the menstruation women susceptible to mild anemia with the symptoms like the pale complexion, listless, cold hands and feet, aversion to cold and sore low back. Eat some raisins every day can avoid those discomfort.

For general health you should try this fantastic food remedy. Soaking one cup of raisins in rice vinegar for 5 days and eat 2 tablespoons of the raisins every morning has amazing therapeutic effects, such as enhance the digestive system and promote metabolism, quickly eliminate fatigue, promote blood circulation, balance blood pressure, improve vision, nourishing blood helps to treat Leukemia and skin disorders, prevent hepatitis, colon cancer, and Alzheimer's disease.

Brown Sugar, White Sugar, and Rock Sugar

Brown sugar, white sugar, and rock sugar all taste sweet and are used for flavor. Most people didn't realize they are not just for flavoring and each one has its own therapeutic effects.

Brown sugar is unrefined sugar. It contains less sugar and rich in nutrients. The therapeutic effects of brown sugar include boost energy, nourish blood and promote blood circulation. For elderly and people with weak constitution can use brown sugar to enhance the immunity. Chinese women drink ginger decoction with brown sugar to treat painful menstruation and clear postpartum lochia after gave birth. Brown sugar is warm in nature. People with warm body constitution and children should eat less. Brown sugar is rich in minerals it shouldn't be cooked for long in order to avoid chemical reaction. For therapeutic purpose the most common way to use brown sugar is to eat with porridge. After the porridge is done add brown sugar.

White sugar is the most commonly used flavor. White sugar is refined sugar and contains much less nutrients than brown sugar. White sugar is cooling in nature and belong to acidic food, excessive consume white sugar is not good for health. White sugar has detoxification effect, can use it to treat seafood poisoning. Drink warm white sugar decoction can cleansing food toxins.

Rock sugar is cooling in nature. It has therapeutic effect of moisten lung and clear lung heat. Drink Chrysanthemum tea with a little rock sugar can clear toxic heat in liver and benefit eyes.

Corn and Corn Silk

Corn is an energy food. Eat corn can strengthen energy. Corn is rich in unsaturated fats especially linoleic acid that helps the metabolism of fat and cholesterol to reduce the deposition of cholesterol in blood vessels and soften arteries. Corn contains natural estrogen. Eat corn can slow down aging process especially for women who are going through menopause. Women add corn in their diet can help to relieve the menopausal symptoms. In Chinese herbal medicine corn silk is listed as an herb. Its therapeutic function affects liver, gallbladder, and urinary bladder channels. The benefits of corn silk include promote urination to relieve urinary tract infection with symptoms of hot and painful urination. It is a natural diuretic. In China people drink corn silk decoction to remove jaundice and lower blood pressure.

How to get the most benefit from corn and corn silk? At supermarket I saw people stripped all corn bran and corn silk when they buy corns. I suggest you take the whole corn home because save the corn bran can keep the moisture and the flavor of the corn. Before you boil the corn you only strip the outside the corn bran and cut off the brown corn silk, keep clean corn bran and corn silk and cook them with the corn can keep the therapeutic effect and the taste. Cook corn for a longer time the better. When the cooking is done you can eat the corn and drink the decoction as tea.

Shan Yao (Chinese Yam)

Chinese Yam is root of the plant. Chinese people call it Shan Yao. In China a lot of fresh Shan Yao sold at farmer's market as vegetable. In the United States we can only buy dried Shan Yao and use it as an herb. Shan Yao is similar to cassava with plain flavor, it is a nutritious food. As an herb Shan Yao plays an important role in Chinese herbal medicine and the raw herb is sold in a form of dried, cut in slices or powder. Therapeutic effects of Shan Yao include enhance digestive system to treat the dysfunction of spleen and stomach. The symptoms include diarrhea, fatigue, lack of appetite, and spontaneous sweating. It is an important ingredient in food therapy for cancer patients, elderly and people in weak constitution. Shan Yao can strengthen immunity and reduce the side effects of chemo therapy. Shan Yao is also beneficial to lung and kidney to treat chronic cough or wheezing due to lung deficiency. To benefit kidney it can treat spermatorrhea, frequent urination, and vaginal discharge which is due to kidney deficiency.

For healthy people having Shan Yao in their diet can boost energy, maintain good health and youth. Shan Yao can cook with rice to make porridge or stir fry to make a dish.

Sweet Potato

Sweet potato is an affordable energy food. It is rich in protein, fatty acid, calcium, iron, and a variety of amino acids. Because sweet potato is nutritious and easy for body to digest and absorb, it is one of the best foods for elderly and frail. Sweet potato contains plenty of carotene which will be converted to Vitamin A, an important vitamin for eyes. Another benefit of sweet potato is moistening intestines to alleviate constipation and prevent colon cancer.

Papaya

Papaya is a tropical fruit. As fruit papaya has delicious taste and as an herb it has unique therapeutic effect that is relaxes sinews. As an herb it benefits liver and spleen. Its therapeutic effects include unblock the channels to clear dampness, release painful obstruction in the joints and the muscles, especially the severe, cramping pain of calve muscles, and strengthening weak lower back and lower extremities. Papaya is the most effective herb for relaxing sinews.

To benefit spleen papaya can harmonize the stomach and eliminate dampness to treat edema. Its anti-inflammatory effect can reduce the swelling of arthritis.

Gan Cao (Licorice Root)

Licorice is not food. I introduce licorice in this book is because when it combines with certain food can make the food very therapeutic. The therapeutic benefits of licorice are harmonizing digestive system, it is commonly used to spleen deficiency with symptoms of heart palpitation that is due to low energy and blood deficiency. The decoction of licorice can be taken internally or applied topically. Drink licorice decoction can moisten lung to treat sore throat and stop coughing. Licorice can alleviate spasms and pain in abdomen or in lower extremities. For external use licorice decoction can clear heat toxicity to treat carbuncles and sores on the skin.

Celery

There is a saying about celery in China. It said that at the beginning celery was used as ornamental plant. After people realized its medicinal value it was listed in the book of material medic as a cooling herb. It has therapeutic effects of soothing liver, clearing toxic heat, promoting urination, and lowering high blood pressure. Because of celery doesn't have any side effects and it is very beneficial to health, it becomes a very popular vegetable. The therapeutic benefits of celery are clear heat, release toxins, and anti-inflammatory.

Remedy for Bad Breath

In case you have bad breath but you don't have dental problem, the bad breath could be caused by food stagnation in stomach or damp-heat in the liver. Every day drink 100ml of fresh celery juice before breakfast and before dinner for one week can treat the cause of this problem.

Remedy for Purify Blood and Brighten Eyes

Ingredients: 50 grams of celery chopped, 15 Gou Qi berries, and 5 dried Chinese dates,

Place all ingredients in a cooking pot. Add 2 cups of water and cook for 20 minutes. Drink the decoction and eat the ingredients once a day for a month. This remedy can lower high blood pressure, eliminate toxins from blood and brighten eyes.

Remedy for Cystitis

Cystitis is a medical term for urinary bladder infection. The symptoms of Cystitis may include pain in pelvic area, or abdomen, or lower back; frequent urination or urgent urination, or difficult urination, or feel burning sensation during urination. If you experience any of these symptoms you can use this remedy.

Mix one cup of chopped celery with three cloves of peeled and smashed garlic in a blender, add a little water and blend it. Remove the dregs and store the juice in a refrigerator. Take the juice twice a day and take 2 tablespoons of the juice each time for 3 to 5 days according to the condition.

While I was writing this book I got bladder infection. At the beginning I didn't realize it was bladder infection. The symptoms I had are difficult urination, lower back pain and stiffness all over the body, especially in the lower extremities. I took an herbal remedy for enhance the function of kidneys for two weeks but the condition was not getting better. Then I realized I made a wrong diagnosis, the cause of the symptoms could be urinary bladder infection. I was glad to have a chance to try this remedy. I took the juice twice a day and each time I took 5 tablespoons of the juice because the taste is not bad at all. Only after took the juice I felt a little discomfort in the stomach because of the garlic. I drank some water and feel fine. The next day I do feel better. The second day I felt much better. On the third day the pain was gone completely. By the way I didn't throw away the dreg, I use them made some pancakes that taste good, too.

Incontinence is also called overactive bladder in the TV commercials. Because of this problem some women use diapers and some had surgeries done on their vaginas. The real cause of the problem is not the dysfunction of urinary bladder or vagina. The urinary bladder loss control is due to kidney Qi (energy) deficiency. This problem can be easily cured by taking Chinese herbal remedy to enhance the function of kidneys or you can use food remedies regularly to keep your kidneys strong and healthy.

Turnip

Turnip can be eaten raw or cooked. Cooked turnip has better therapeutic effects. The water that used to cook the turnip is very therapeutic, too. For symptoms such as indigestion caused by food stagnation, stomach bloating, no appetite, and constipation, drink turnip decoction can treat those symptoms.

For young Children with poor digestion and internal heat that lead to symptoms like hot palms, irritability, red face and dry lips, with this kind of physical constitution the young kids will get common cold and flu easily. Add some rock sugar in the turnip decoction can clear internal heat quickly and the young kids will love the taste of the drink. Drink the decoction 2 to 3 times a day for a couple of days can release the symptoms and prevent common cold and flu.

Turnip decoction has good benefit to lung. For people with asthma and chronic cough with sputum, drink turnip decoction without sugar everyday can improve the condition. Or use 1000 grams of turnip squeeze the juice and add 2 tablespoons of honey in the juice. Store the juice in a refrigerator. Take the juice 3 times a day and each time take one table spoon of the juice can get significant improvement in a week.

Scientific research found turnip contains a substance that has the anti-tumor and antiviral effects, and it has significant inhibit effect on certain cancer cells, such as esophageal cancer cell, nasal cancer cell, and uterus cancer cell. In order to make this substance fully released from the turnip patient need eat raw turnip and take more time to chew the turnip well. Every day or every the other day eat 100-150 grams of raw turnip. Over eating of raw turnip may have side effect.

Remedy for Migraine Headache

Squeeze some turnip juice set aside. Let the patient lie down on his back. Fold a towel and put it under the patient's neck in order to make his head slightly upturned. If the patient's headache is on the left side of the head, implant a few drops of turnip juice in his right nostril. If the headache is on the right side, implant a few drops of turnip juice into the left nostril. Use this natural therapy can release migraine headache in five minutes. You can use a straw to collect turnip juice if you don't have the right tool.

Remedy for Foot Odor and Foot Sweat

Another therapeutic effect of turnip is clearing dampness and killing bacteria. Use turnip decoction soak feet can treat Beriberi, sweat feet, swollen feet, and eliminate foot odor. Cut turnip in slices and cook in boiling water for 15 minutes; remove the turnip and use the decoction soak feet. Use this therapy once a day for 15 days the problem can be solved.

Remedy for Hemorrhoids

Turnip also can be used to treat hemorrhoids. Cut one big turnip (or 4 small turnips) into slices and place them in a cooking pot, add half gallon of water cooking for 10 minutes. Remove the turnip and use the decoction wash the affected area. The same decoction can be used for three times. Keep the decoction in a refrigerator for next day use. The next day warm up the decoction before to use. After the decoction has been used three times make the new decoction. Use this remedy every day for 20 days.

Black Fungus and White Fungus

In western culture most people have not seen black fungus and white fungus. They are popular food in eastern countries because of their therapeutic effects. Both black fungus and white fungus grow from trunks of the trees. Black fungus contains vitamin B1, B2, iron, Carotene, Lecithin, Cephaline, and calcium. It has the benefits of anti-thrombotic (eliminate blood clots), prevent cardiovascular diseases, improve the quality of blood, boost energy, enhance immunity, and prevent cancer. Black fungus contains a substance called AAP that can lower blood glucose, lower LDL cholesterol, and heal ulcers. AAP can be easily affected by high temperature therefore cook black fungus for a longer time could destroy AAP. The correct way of cooking black fungus is soaking a few of them in cold water for one hour. After dried black fungus socked in water they will expend and become fresh black fungus. In order to avoid the nutrients dissolved in water, do not soak black fungus in water for more than 2 hours. You can stir fried socked black fungus with other vegetables, or cook them in boiling water for 5 minutes and mixed with other vegetable to make salad.

White fungus has the benefits of moistening lung to stop dry cough, relieve dry mouth, hot flashes, constipation, irritability, and insomnia. Like black fungus when soaked in water dried white fungus will expend and become fresh white fungus. Many people after age 50 experience the dryness like dry throat, dry mouth and dry cough. Soak half white fungus in cold water for an hour and cook in boiling water for 40 to 60 minutes. After turn off the heat add some rock sugar and some Gou Qi berries. Drink the decoction and eat the ingredients, you will get relief on the same day.

Kelp (Seaweed)

Kelp is a very popular food in Japanese food culture and it is also listed in Chinese herbal medicine as an herb because of its therapeutic effects which include promote urination to eliminate edema and tumor, and enhance the immunity. Kelp contains large amount of iodine that can stimulate the pituitary gland to restore the normal function of the ovarian and keep endocrine balanced to prevent breast hyperplasia. Kelp is also beneficial to people with hypertension and high cholesterol. Kelp is rich in unsaturated fatty acids that can help to reduce blood viscosity and prevent the hardening of the arteries.

Kelp is rich in fiber. It is a low fat and low calorie food. Japan is a longevity country and Japanese people consider kelp as a longevity food. It is said many people in Japan at very old age can keep good vision, sharp mind, and physically active is the result of eating Zen Soup (Miso soup). Zen Soup is made of kelp and bean curd.

Contraindication:

1. Patients with hyperthyroidism do not eat kelp. The iodine in kelp can make their condition worse.

2. Pregnant women and breastfeeding women should not eat kelp in order to avoid iodine get into fetus and baby's body to cause thyroid dysfunction.

Zen Soup Recipe

Soak 60 grams of dried kelp in cold water over night. Wash it clean and cut into small pieces. 250 grams of bean curd cut into small cubes. One green onion finely cut.

Cook kelp in boiling water for 30 minutes, add one tablespoon of Miso paste and bean curd into the soup, cook for 5 minutes more. After turn off the heat add the green onion in it.

Chapter Three

Natural Remedies for Self Cure

Remedy for Headache and Toothache

To treat headache squeeze 10ml of fresh ginger juice, add one teaspoon of sesame oil and one teaspoon of honey in the juice. Stir the mixture well. Apply the mixture on headache site.

To treat Migraine headache, cut two slices of radish with skin. Stick the radish on temple area and fix them with bandage for 20 minutes.

To treat toothache grind a small piece of fresh ginger in a blender and add little flour into grinded ginger to make paste and stick the paste on painful side of the face. This remedy is only for temperate relieve.

Remedy for Glaucoma

Glaucoma is a serious eye disease. Based on scientific study Glaucoma is due to certain eye structural defects cause increased eye pressure and can lead to blindness. I have treated several Glaucoma cases, all those cases after 1 or 2 treatment sessions the patients' eye pressure reading decreased to the normal range but to improve their vision is very difficult. One case is a 68-year-old woman with congenital Glaucoma. She almost lost all her vision. Both of her eyes pressure reading is over 20. After the first session I got an email from her in late afternoon. In the email she said after lunch she took a nap when she woke up she saw everything in front of her is clear. Sounds like a miracle happened but I was wondering how long her vision can be last. Next day I called her. She told me after she woke up from the nap she saw everything was so clear, she was so happy and she went to the theater watched a movie then she lost her vision again. After the third session she went to see her eye doctor and both of her eyes pressure reading dropped down to 9. She told me her doctor said 9 is the normal reading. For people with Glaucoma get adequate sleep and avoid long time watching TV or using computer are very important. Long-term of using painkillers also can lead to increased intraocular pressure.

About Glaucoma western medical study has been limited on the disorder of the eye. Chinese medicine is holistic medicine, according to Chinese medicine theory certain eye disorders are connected to the disorders of the liver and emotions of upset, depress, and rage that could cause the heat accumulation in the liver and liver Qi stagnation. Actually many health issues are related to unbalanced emotions, such as digestion disorders, depression, hypertension, and stroke, etc. People with Glaucoma remain a calm state of mind is very important. Don't look for other people's fault. Don't blame others if something went wrong. Personality does affect a person's health and all aspects of his life. There is a saying that people are divided into three ranks. The finest people have the capability and have no temper. The moderate people have the capability and the temper. The low-grade people have no capability but the temper. What kind of person you want to be? I consider myself is belong to the moderate people and try to improve myself.

This remedy needs one ingredient - sunflower. Get a big sunflower and have the seeds removed. Cut the sunflower to smaller pieces and cook the ingredient in one gallon boiling water for 20 minutes. Then remove the ingredient from the water and use the decoction steam the eyes first. When the decoction is still warm use it to wash eyes. Use this treatment once a day. The decoction can be saved in a fridge for the next day use. The next day warm up the decoction before to use and the same decoction can be used for 3 times.

Remedy for Improving Vision

This remedy is for improving near sighted eye disorder or weak vision. The cause of this kind of eye disorder is due to the insufficiency of liver blood and kidney essence. The function of liver is cleansing blood and store blood. The symptoms of liver blood deficiency may have other symptoms which include vertigo, dizziness, dry and irritating sensation in the eyes, blurred vision, and night blindness.

Soak 50 grams of black beans in cold water for 4 hours. Place the soaked black beans and 50 grams of dried Chinese dates in a cooking pot, add two cups of water cook for 30 minutes. Turn off the heat and add 30 grams wolfberries. Eat the ingredients once a day as desert for a week you will notice the improvement of the vision.

To treat night blindness and vision loss, use 6 grams of wolfberries and 6 grams chrysanthemum to make tea. Drink the tea often can improve the vision.

Remedy for Cataract

Cataract is an aging related eye disorder. Almost everyone reach age of 40 will gradually develop the symptoms of Cataract. Like other health issues preventing of Cataract is easier than cure it. Keep using this remedy can keep your vision sharp for the rest of your life.

Put two tablespoons of white vinegar in a large bowl and filled the bowl with very hot water. Use the water steam the eyes first, when the water cools down use the water wash the eyes and the face. Vinegar can promote blood circulation. Keep using this remedy every day for a while you will notice the improvement of the vision and the condition of the skin.

Remedy for Nourishing Liver and Brighten Eyes

Cut a pear to some pieces and put them in a small bowl. Add two tablespoons of vinegar in the bowl. Eat one pear a day will have the benefits of eliminating the symptoms of dry mouth, bitter taste in the mouth, insomnia, irritability that is due to liver yin deficiency (dryness and heat in the liver). Also improve the condition of the eyes, such as dry eyes, red or swollen eyes, and blurred vision.

Remedy for Toothache

Put 50 grams of Beehive in a cooking pot, add 3 cups of water cook over high heat until water is boiling turn to low heat until the water is reduced by half, turn off the heat and add 50 grams of brown sugar. Drink the whole decoction that can make you toothache free for ten years.

Here is another way to treat toothache. Use a cotton ball dip some honey first, then dip some base powder， press the cotton ball on the painful tooth for five minutes, can relief the pain. This remedy can be used to stop all kinds of toothache. Plus use green tea rinse the mouth several times a day.

Remedy for Gum Bleeding

Ingredient: 5 grams of peanuts with red skin, two cups of vinegar. Soak the peanuts in the vinegar for two days. Use the vinegar to rinse month. Keep the vinegar in the mouth for three minutes. Use this remedy twice a day for five days the gum bleeding will be cured.

Remedy for Cardiovascular Disorders

To prevent cardiovascular disorders many people taking prescription drugs sometimes the side effects of the drugs can be more dangerous than cardiovascular disease itself. Actually to treat cardiovascular diseases there are some very good herbal remedies are available in Chinese medicine for strengthening the function of heart, promote blood circulation of the heart and without any side effects.

This remedy can soften blood vessels, lower high blood pressure, lower LDL cholesterol level, and promote blood flow of the heart. Keep using this food remedy you can quit prescription drugs.

Ingredients: 250 grams peanuts with red skin, a bottle of vinegar

Put the peanuts in a glass jar and add vinegar into the jar until it covers the peanuts. Seal the jar and keep it in a refrigerator for a week. Every day eat 7 to 10 peanuts in the evening. Do not over eat the peanuts. Keep using this remedy and check your blood pressure, if the blood pressure reading is normal, keep using the remedy and gradually reducing the medication.

Remedy for High Blood Viscosity

Blood viscosity is a measure of the thickness of blood. Scientific studies discovered some high blood pressure cases are due to high blood viscosity. When blood viscosity decrease will make blood flow more smooth and reduce blood pressure. You may use this natural remedy to improve the quality of your blood.

Ingredients: one pound of fresh ginger after washed clean cut into thin slices, half pound of rock sugar, and a bottle of rice vinegar

Put thin sliced ginger, rock sugar and rice vinegar into a glass jar. Cover the jar and leave it in the room temperature for a week then it is ready to use. Every morning eat 5 to 8 slices of ginger and drink one tablespoon of the vinegar before breakfast. (Do not eat in the evening. Eat ginger in the morning can boost energy, eat ginger in the evening is harmful.) After finished the whole jar of the ginger the blood viscosity should be reduced to the normal level. When you are using this remedy if you experience the symptoms like dry mouth or sweat, you can drink a small glass of honey water every day to eliminate the symptoms.

Remedy for Opening Blocked Arteries

I was told no matter how badly the arteries blocked with this natural remedy they can be opened quickly. This remedy was passed down in a family for several generations. A 64-year-old man was diagnosed with three heart arteries are seriously blocked and a triple bypass surgery was scheduled in three weeks. While he was preparing money for the surgery he got this remedy and used it every day. Before his surgery the final test result showed that all of his arteries are opened and clean. The surgery was canceled and his money was saved.

Ingredients: One cup of lemon juice, one cup of fresh ginger juice, one cup of apple vinegar, one whole garlic peeled and smashed to paste, and two tablespoons of honey

In a cooking pot mix the lemon juice, ginger juice, apple vinegar and garlic paste together and cook the mixed juices over medium heat until the juice is boiling change to low heat continue cook for 15 minutes. After turned off the heat waiting for the decoction cools down, then add two tablespoons of honey in the decoction and stir it even. Put the decoction in a glass bottle and store it in a refrigerator. Each day take one tablespoon of the decoction before the breakfast until finish the whole bottle of the decoction. Make an appointment with your doctor to check your arteries. Using this remedy can balance blood pressure. Check your blood pressure if the blood pressure reading is low you need reduce or stop taking lower blood pressure medication.

Remedies for Kidney Disorders

Remedy for Uremia

Uremia is a serious and complicated kidney disorder and acute renal failure. It occurs when kidneys are unable to eliminate urea and other waste products from the body. In western medicine practice kidney dialysis is the treatment being used to relieve the symptoms and for most cases kidney transplant are needed. In Chinese medicine the treatment combine with certain herbal remedies can treat uremia effectively. One case in my own practice, a 54-year-old woman with uremia came to see me for severe lower back pain and she told me soon she will start dialysis treatment. She is open-minded to alternative medicine. I used massage, cupping therapy, Moxibustion therapy in her treatment sessions. After four sessions her creatinine dropped from 1300 to 880 and she regained the sensation of holding the urine, and both the force of urination and the volume of the urine are increased.

Most uremia patients have no idea how their kidneys were damaged so badly. In many cases when our internal organs, such as heart, lung, liver, and kidneys are damaged we don't feel pain, therefore once a person realized he need medical attention his condition is already at the late stage of the disease. Uremia is one of those cases. What is the cause of the uremia and how to prevent it? Kidney is a very vulnerable organ, the following mistakes you should try to avoid in order to protecting your kidneys.

1. Long-term stay up late can cause the damage to liver and kidneys. You must lie down and rest to allow your body to produce kidney essence and for the liver to does purify the blood work. Go to bed no later than 11pm.

2. Long-term taking medication especially many people use painkiller to manage pain that have the site effects on the kidneys.

3. Over taking supplements such as protein can cause burden on kidneys.

4. High-intensity physical exertion and mental work, stress, over thinking, and worry can deplete kidney essence.

5. Excessive consume alcohol and indulge sex life can cause kidney deficiency.

6. Over consuming greasy food and strong flavored food, the food that is too salty, too sweet, or too much protein can increase the burden on kidneys.

7. Eat seafood with beer could produce too much uric acid and urea nitrogen that could lead to Hyperuricemia, kidney stones and uremia.

This folk remedy has no record to show how many people were cured by using it. One real case is a uremia patient with full body edema was discharged from a hospital. His doctor's prognosis was he only has one to two weeks to live. His family got this remedy from a relative. When the family saw the remedy they doubted it can help because only two ingredients are needed and both of them are food. They made the remedy for him and they didn't expect the healing started immediately. After the patient ate that porridge (What they made just like a meal.) he urinated a lot and there was bloodshot in his urine. He kept on using this remedy for a month and his uremia was cured.

Ingredients: ½ cup of Mung beans (Chinese green beans), a whole garlic pilled and crashed

Put 3 cups of water in a cooking pot cook over high heat. When the water is boiling add the Mung beans and the garlic in boiling water cook over low heat for 30 minutes. After turn off the heat add a little salt for flavor. Eat as a meal twice a day. Actually because the ingredients are foods there is no strict requirement about the amount of the ingredients. I give a measurement for you to have an idea, eat more or less there is no side effects at all.

Remedy for Enhance the Function of Kidney

A man was suffering from Rheumatoid arthritis that also affected on other internal organs particularly his kidneys were severely damaged. In a hospital he was told by his doctor that his kidney's condition soon will develop to Uremia but there was no treatment available to control the condition. A relative gave him a folk remedy that only needs two ingredients peanuts and Chinese dried dates. He thought if this remedy doesn't work it won't cause any problem by eating peanuts and Dates. He started using this remedy once a day. On the third day the swollen of his legs started to subside. He continued using this remedy for another two weeks and his uremia was cured. This remedy is very effective for strengthening the function of the kidneys, and it can be used for other kidney disorders as well.

Ingredients: 60 grams dried Chinese dates, 60 grams peanuts with red skin

Cook the dates and the peanuts in boiling water until the ingredients are well cooked. Eat the ingredients with the decoction as breakfast.

Remedy for Kidney Stones

Except to eliminate kidney stones and urinary tract stones this remedy also can be used to lower blood pressure, Clean toxic heat, calm down irritability, and treat the symptoms of dry mouth or ulcer in the mouth.

Cut a fresh gourd into ½ inches dice and cook in boiling water for 10 minutes. After turn off the heat add some rock sugar and divided the remedy into two equal parts. Eat one part in the morning and eat the other half in the evening every day for 15 days.

A Dish for Impotence

Impotence is generally due to the exhaustion of kidney essence and kidney Qi deficiency from indulgent sexual activity and excessive masturbation. Except the failure of making erection or weak erection, impotent patient also could experience other symptoms, such as the pain or weakness in lower back and legs, emission, cold extremities, dizziness, spontaneous sweating, frequent urination, and enuresis. Using Viagra or other erectile enhancers can cause further damage to the kidneys. To treat impotence the approach of Chinese medicine is using therapies and herbal remedies to reinforce the function of the kidney. During the treatment about two months the patient should eat well, resting well and avoid smoking, drinking alcohol and having sex, the function of kidney can be restored.

This is a very popular dish in Chinese cooking culture. Eat this dish often can enhance the function of kidney and replenish kidney essence.

Ingredients: 250 grams of shrimp shelled, 200 grams of chives chopped, a small piece of fresh ginger shredded, cooking wine, and salt

Put a pan over a medium heat and add 2 tablespoons of cooking oil in the pan. When the oil getting hot put in shredded ginger stir fry for one minute, put in shrimp stir fry for two minutes, add a little cooking wine stir and add in chives, salt stir fry for one minute turn off the heat. It is done.

For both men and women must keep their kidney healthy to enjoy sex. According to Chinese medicine theory that excessive mental work or labor work, and excessive sexual activity all can weaken the kidney. Here is a real case.

One Saturday afternoon, a 30-year-old woman with severe lower back pain and other kidney deficiency symptoms came to see me. After the treatment she felt much better. When she was leaving I said to her "tell your husband no sex for two weeks." She laughed. After the weekend she called on Monday morning said her lower back getting worse again and made an appointment for more treatment. Later she told me on Sunday she felt no pain at all then they had sex.

Remedies for Digestion Disorders

Remedy for Esophageal Spasm

The symptoms of Esophageal Spasm may include pain in the chest, sometimes the pain is so intense which could be mistaken for heart pain (angina). The patient can have a feeling that an object is stuck in the throat, regurgitation, and have difficulty to swallow food. According to Chinese medicine theory the real cause of esophageal spasm is due to emotional stress or stomach and spleen Qi deficiency. Ginger can strengthen stomach Qi and spleen Qi and promote Qi circulation.

Place 5 grams of ginger powder and 3 slices of fresh ginger in a mug, add boiling water to make hot tea. Drink this ginger tea daily for a week, the spasm can be cured.

Remedy for Food Poisoning

Cook 50 grams of licorice and 100 grams of Mung beans together in boiling water for 20 minutes. Remove the licorice drink the decoction and eat the mung beans for detoxification.

Remedy for Abdominal Pain

There are different disorders can cause abdominal pain. This remedy is very effective for abdominal pain caused by cold accumulation in stomach or in intestines. Overeating raw food or cold food can cause cold accumulation in digestive system. The symptoms include stomachache and abdominal pain, bloating, and loose or watery stool. This remedy does not help with abdominal pain that is due to Appendicitis or gynecologic disorders.

Cut 250 grams of white turnip to slices and put in a cooking pot, add 5 slices of ginger and 5 cups of water. Cook over high heat until water is boiling turn to the low heat cook for 15 minutes. After turn off the heat add a little salt and pepper for flavor. Eat the soup when it is very warm can get immediate relief of the pain.

Remedy for Gallstones, Diabetes, and Quit Smoking

If where you live close to a pumpkin farm you can get the ingredient of this remedy free. This remedy can cure gallstones, kidney stones, and Diabetes. Use this remedy also can quit smoking in seven days. What you need is the pumpkin vine and leaves. Collect some pumpkin vines and leaves, wash them clean and cut the vine and leaves to small pieces. Put the ingredient at a place that is cooling with good ventilation and wait for them to dry. After they completely dried you can store them in a container. Each time take 100-150 grams of pumpkin leaves and cook them in one gallon of boiling water for five minutes. Remove the leaves and add a little brown sugar, drink this decoction as tea every day. During the time of using this remedy do not eat greasy and spicy food, do not smocking, do not drinking alcohol, otherwise invalid.

For kidney stones and gallbladder stones, after drinking the decoction 4 to 5 days the small particles and powder start to discharge from urethra. On the 6th or 7th day will have sticky urine discharged that indicates all stones have been melted and discharged. In most cases after drinking the decoction for seven days the patient's CT result will show he is stone free.

For quit smoking, drink the decoction every day for 7 days. After the person drank the decoction for 7 days, he doesn't want to smock any more.

Remedy for Constipation

This remedy is for external application. Prepare a small piece of ginger finely chopped, vinegar, alcohol, and a bandage. In this application the purpose of the alcohol use is not for disinfection, it is used as a guiding herb, and it will guide the ginger's therapeutic effect into the kidneys to promote the kidney metabolism. The function of the vinegar is to soften the stools.

First using a cotton ball soak in alcohol and rub on the belly button. Fill the belly button with the ginger and apply two drops of vinegar on the ginger, use the bandage to cover the belly button. Apply this remedy before go to sleep. Next day if the constipation is alleviated you can remove the ginger. If the constipation has not been alleviated keep the ginger in the belly button for 24 hours. Usually the constipation will be completely released in less than three days.

There are different causes for constipation. Sometimes you need try different remedies and find the one that works for you.

*Vinegar is rich in amino acids also contains lots of digestive enzymes that can promote the movement of intestines. In the morning before to have breakfast prepare a glass of warm water, add one teaspoon of honey and ten drops of vinegar and stir. Drinking the water with empty stomach for one week can promote bowel movement and clean up the intestines.

*In the morning before the breakfast drinking a teaspoon of sesame oil with warm water can release constipation the same day.

*Peel one potato and squeeze potato juice. Drink potato juice twice a day. Drink once in the morning with empty stomach and drink one time after lunch.

*Every day eat 15g of pine nuts and avoid eat spicy food.

Remedy for Hemorrhoids

Many people suffering Hemorrhoids for decades couldn't find cure. Except the discomfort of itching and pain, frequent or excessive bleeding can cause stress, dizziness, and vertigo. Using this remedy many Hemorrhoids patients were cured in couple of weeks.

A 60 year-old man had hemorrhoids for more than 20 years didn't find cure. Frequent bleeding lead to anemia and cause him dizziness and vertigo. He was cured by using this remedy. Prepare two cups of warm water and add 2 tablespoon of glucose. Drink the water twice a day, before breakfast and before dinner. After he finished one bag of glucose (500 grams) he was cured without recurrence.

Remedy for Acid Reflux

Acid reflux is a very common seen problem in people at age over 50. In some serious cases patients feel the heat and pain in stomach and esophagus. The cause of this problem is unknown to western medical study. Many patients were treated with surgeries. According to Chinese medicine theory this problem is due to stomach and spleen Qi (energy) deficiency. A Chinese herbal remedy called Gui Pi Wan treat this problem very effective and without any side effects. A 72-year-old woman came to see me for neck pain. At the end of the session she said her neck problem is due to acid reflux that she had suffered for more than 20 years. In order to avoid the acid fluid moving upward she sleeps almost in a sitting position that lead to the pain of her neck. I suggest she take Chinese herbal remedy Gui Pi Wan. After she took a few bottles of the remedy her acid reflux problem was gone and she felt her energy is much better. Gui Pi Wan is a very commonly used remedy in Chinese medicine clinics. Gui Pi Wan is used to strengthen the function of spleen. Spleen is an important organ which responsible for metabolism in digestive system. Many people especially women after 50 their metabolism slow down that can cause symptoms like acid reflux, stomach bloating after meal, gaining weight, water retention, low energy, plus blood deficiency symptoms, such as dry skin, dry hair, and losing hair. Gui Pi Wan treats the cause and the symptoms. If you cannot find the remedy you can use baking soda for temperate relieve.

Put 0.5g of baking soda in a glass, add 200cc hot water and stir to make baking soda dissolved in the water. Drink the baking soda water slowly, when stomach acid mixed with baking soda will generate Carbon dioxide gas that will release from the mouth and acid reflux can be eased immediately. This is a way for temperate release the symptom.

Remedy for Stomach Ulcer

The main ingredient of this remedy is 15 chicken eggshells. Bake eggshells over low heat until they turned to light brown. Grind the baked eggshells into fine powder and set aside. Use a saucepan bake 120g flour over low heat until the flour turned to light yellow. Mix the flour and the eggshell powder together, add two tablespoons of sugar and mix well. Store the powder in a jar. Take this remedy twice a day before the meals. Each time put half tablespoon of the powder in a bowl add a little boiling water to make the paste. After finished all the powder the stomach ulcer should be healed.

Remedy for Gout

People with Gout strictly control diet is very important. Gout is due to the Purine metabolism disorder that leads to uric acid in the blood increased. The symptoms of Gout include a sudden burning pain that is almost unbearable, swollen and painful joints typically found in big toe with redness and swelling. Gout also can affect the joints of feet, ankles, knees, hands and wrists. The affected joints are often stiff and difficult to bend. The following are some natural remedies for treating Gout.

1. Take one raw potato peeled and cut to small pieces and put in a blender, add one cup of pure cranberry juice in the blender blend the ingredients to make the smoothies. Drink one cup of the smoothies a day. Pain can be released in 1 to 2 days. Keep using this remedy Gout can be cured in 10 to 15 days.

2. Mix 5g Cinnamon powder with some honey and eat it once a day. Meanwhile eat more greens and unpolished grains.

3. People with Gout suffering inflammation in joints and muscle tissues that is caused by accumulation of toxic heat in the body. Radish has the therapeutic effects of clear heat, release the toxins, clear mucus and stop coughing. Eat raw radish everyday also can improve the condition of Gout.

Remedies for Respiratory Disorders

Remedies for Common Cold, Flu, and Cough

Common cold and Flu are very popular diseases that affect people at all ages. At flu season it is very easy to get it at public places, and when one person got it can make the whole family sick. Here is a tip to prevent flu spread in your home. Put 1/3 cup of vinegar in a small sauce pan and cook it over medium heat until the vinegar is boiling, cook a few minutes more let the smell filled the house. This is a natural way to kill bacterial and prevent common cold and flu.

Soup Recipe for Common Cold

This is the most commonly used remedy to treat common cold by Chinese people. Cut 5 slices of fresh ginger, 3 green onions only use white part with root, 2 cloves of garlic pilled and crashed. Put all the ingredients in boiling water cook for two minutes. After turn off heat add a teaspoon of dark brown sugar and drink the decoction like hot tea. Keep yourself warm to let yourself sweat a little bit. Cold will expel from your body so as the toxins. Have a good night sleep the next day you should feel fine.

Remedy for Chronic Cough

Cut 7 pieces thinly sliced ginger. Put a tablespoon of sesame oil (Use other kind of oil will not get the same result.) in a saucepan and put in sliced ginger fry over low heat until the ginger turned to light yellow. Dip the ginger with a little white sugar when you eat. For mild condition you can get relief immediately. Keep using this remedy once a day for three days the cough can be cured completely. For chronic cough keep using this remedy for seven days.

Remedy for Cure Asthma (1)

Ingredients: 100 grams of sesame seeds, 250 grams of walnuts, one tablespoon of honey

Grind sesame seeds and walnuts to fine powder, mix the powder together. Put two tablespoons of water and one tablespoon of honey in a saucepan, cook over medium heat till the water is boiling add the mixed powder into the saucepan stir fry until smell the aroma. Remove the powder into a bowl and put the bowl in a steamer to steam for 30 minutes. Wait for the powder cools down then transfer it into a container and store it in a refrigerator.

Everyday take one tablespoon of the remedy in the morning and take one tablespoon in the evening. Asthma can be completely cured in three to six months.

Remedy for Cure Asthma (2)

Ingredients: 2 walnuts chopped to smaller pieces, in a small bowl whisk 2 chicken eggs, some rock sugar

Put walnuts in a cooking pot and add 2 cups of water. Cook the walnuts in boiling water for 5 minutes and slowly pour whisked eggs into the boiling water and turn off the heat. Add little rock sugar in it. Eat this soup every day before breakfast. The symptoms will be gone in ten days.

Turnip Tea for Chronic Cough

Use a medium sized white turnip, wash it clean and cut into 1/2 inch dices, place the turnip in a glass jar and fill about 2/3 of the jar with turnip, then add the honey into the jar until the honey covers the turnip. Close the jar and store it in a refrigerator for overnight, the next day take 2 tablespoons of the liquid and some turnip put into a cup and fill the cup with very hot water. Drink as hot tea twice a day. Drink the tea every day for seven days the chronic cough can be cured.

A Simple Therapy for Clod and Cough

This natural therapy is very simple everyone can learn how to do it. Actually this therapy can treat more than cold and cough. When the treatment performed on upper back area and shoulders can expel cold and stop coughing, promote blood circulation and improve the function of lung and heart. If the treatment performed on middle part of the back can benefit digestive system to treat food stagnation and poor digestion. If the treatment performed on lower back area can benefit kidneys and relieve lower back pain.

Take a large size of fresh ginger root finely chopped and mixed with 2 tablespoons of cooking oil to make the paste. Put the paste in a microwave to warm it up. Put the warm ginger paste on the patient's upper back and massage the back, the shoulders, and the neck. Or use a piece of cloth wrap the ginger paste in the cloth and tied it up. Put the wrapped ginger in a microwave to warm it up. Hold the wrapped ginger massage on the back or the painful area. This way you can warm up the ginger paste repeatedly and work on different area.

Remedies for Foot and Nails

Remedies for Beriberi (Athlete's foot)

Athlete's foot is a common name for a fungal infection of the foot. Put 100 grams of green tea in a plastic basin and add 2000-3000ml boiling water in the basin, soak the feet with the warm decoction for 15 to 30 minutes. Keep soaking the feet once a day for 3 days. For serious condition may need 5 days for Beriberi to be cured. Once the infection was cured it will not have recurrence. Do not use metal basin.

Another remedy will cost you nothing if you can find a willow tree. Collect 50g of fresh leaves from a willow tree. Cut the leaves to small pieces and put them in your socks, wear the socks to sleep during the night. You will see improvement the next morning. Keep using this remedy for 3 to 4 days beriberi can be cured.

Remedies for Foot Odor

Add 10 to 15ml of vinegar in half gallon of hot water and use the water soaking the feet for 15 minutes. Soak the feet once a day for 3 to 4 days can eliminate foot odor.

Or cook some fresh ginger in boiling water for 10 minutes then remove the ginger and add a little salt in the ginger decoction. Use the ginger decoction soak feet can eliminate foot odor and relieve fatigue.

Remedy for Nail Fungus

If you get fungal infection in fingernails or toenails that cause the thickening, roughness, and splitting of the nails you can apply some vinegar into fungal infected nails. Apply several times a day the infection can be cured quickly. Vinegar also can make the new nails shine.

I shared this remedy with a cancer patient. She had fungal infection in her toenails, her toenails turned thick and yellow that was the result of side effects of chemotherapy. According to Chinese medicine theory the nails condition reflect the condition of liver. Chemotherapy left toxins in liver and reflected on nails as fungal infection. Her toenails turned thick and yellow. She tried this simple remedy and was amazed by the result. The fungus infection completely disappeared in one week.

Or smash 100g of garlic and soak the garlic in one bottle of vinegar for one day. Use the vinegar soaking the hands and feet.

Remedies for Sleeping Disorders

Remedy for Insomnia

Insomnia is a very commonly seen health issue. At my work very often hear people say "I always wake up during the night or it is difficult for me to fall asleep, maybe I need to change my mattress." Some people with neck or shoulder pain also say that their pain maybe caused by their pillows. I ask them one question "If you got constipated are you going to change your toilet?" Insomnia is caused by many factors. There are disease factors, physiological factors, and psychological factors. If your body doesn't affect by any of those factors you will sleep like a baby.

The leaves on peanut plants, the shell of peanut, and the red skin of peanut all have therapeutic effects. The shell of peanuts can promote blood circulation, soften the vines and arteries. Put some peanut shells in a cup and pour in boiling water to make hot tea and drink the tea regularly can prevent cardiovascular diseases. Red skin of peanut has the function of replenishing blood. The leaves of the peanut plant have the effects of calm down the mind and treat insomnia. Wash a handful of fresh or dried peanut leaves clean and cook them in 250ml of boiling water for 5 minutes and drink the decoction as hot tea. Drink one cup of the tea in the morning and drink one cup of the tea in the evening, keep drinking this tea for at least 15 days.

Remedy for Insomnia

This remedy is for the people who suffering insomnia with the symptoms, such as irritability, dry mouth, over-thinking, toss and turn having difficulty to fall asleep. There is a new ingredient in this remedy called Bai He, translate in English is Lily bulb. In Chinese herbal medicine Bai He is listed as a top grade herb without any side effects. In China fresh Bai He are sold at farmer's market and people use them to cook dish. Dried Bai He is usually cooked with rice to make porridge. Here in the United States dried Bai He sold at Chinese supermarkets. In some Chinese herbal remedies Bai He is used for cleansing the toxic heat, moistening the lung to treat dry cough, and calms the spirit to treat the symptoms of insomnia, irritability, restlessness, and heart palpitation.

Ingredients: 25 grams of Bai He, 25 grams of Mung beans, one cup of milk

Soak Bai He and Mung beans in cold water for 2 hours. Put soaked ingredients in boiling water and cook over low heat for 45 minutes. After turn off the heat add a little rock sugar and milk. Milk contains Tryptophan which can transform to Serotonin, Serotonin can promote sleep. You can have this delicious remedy as dessert after dinner.

Remedy for Chronic Insomnia

Chronic insomnia is not a disease but a symptom. People suffering chronic insomnia may also have other symptoms, such as restlessness, anxiety, over thinking, dry skin, dry hair even losing hair, and difficult fall asleep at night but feel very sleepy during the day especially when they are driving. In this case the cause of insomnia could be due to blood deficiency. If the cause not being treated the condition cannot be improved. This remedy has two ingredients Chinese dried dates and ginger. Chinese dried date nourishes blood and ginger promotes blood circulation. By improving the condition of blood can solve the problem of insomnia.

One tablespoon of fresh mince ginger and ten dried dates together put in a small cooking pot and add one cup of water cook over medium heat until the water is boiling turn to low heat cook for 10 minutes more. Turn off the heat add a little salt and sesame oil. Eat the whole thing when it is warm. Eat with breakfast for about one month the condition should be improved.

Remedy for Poor Sleep with Dreams

Ingredients: 50 grams of Chi Xiao Dou (Chinese red beans), 50 grams shells of peanuts, 50 grams of wheat kernels

Soak 50 grams of Chi Xiao Dou in cold water for one hour. Cook all ingredients together in 1000ml boiling water for 30 minutes. Remove the shells of peanut and add some honey. Eat one time in the morning and another time in the evening for 5 to 7 days the condition will be improved.

Remedies for Skin Disorders

Remedy for Psoriasis (1)

This remedy can treat Psoriasis, Shingles, and the inflammation of the skin. Place an egg in a small bowl (with the shell) and add vinegar into the bowl until the vinegar covered the egg. Soak the egg in vinegar for one week. After one week take the egg out of the vinegar, break the egg shell and put egg white and yolk in a clean bowl. Use a cotton ball dip in the egg white and apply it on affected area. Use this remedy once a day until the symptoms subside.

Remedy for Psoriasis (2)

This remedy can be used to cure Psoriasis, Shingles, itchy skin and inflamed skin condition. A man who shared this remedy suffered Psoriasis for more than 20 years and spent a lot of money didn't find cure until he got this remedy his Psoriasis was cured.

Ingredients: One bottle of white vinegar, 20 grams of Hua Jiao (Hua Jiao is red pepper. It looks like black pepper but in color red. It is sold at Chinese supermarkets.)

Cook vinegar and Hua Jiao together in a cooking pot for 30 minutes. After the vinegar cools down, remove the Hua jiao from vinegar, put the vinegar in a spray bottle and spray it on the affected skin. Or use a cotton ball dip the vinegar and apply it on affected skin 3 times a day until the skin disorder is cured. The result of this remedy is fantastic.

One day one of my patients called and told me she got Shingles. She couldn't come to see me because the shingles was so painful even putting on her clothes will cause more pain. I told her have her son come to pick up a remedy. I prepared the remedy and put it back in vinegar bottle. The next day she called me in the morning "Gina, what's in that remedy? I tried many remedies nothing helps. This remedy stops the pain right away."

Remedy for Persistent Psoriasis

Cut 250 grams of chives to ½ inch long and put them in a saucepan bake over low heat until they are completely dried. Grind baked chives to powder and mix with some lard. Apply the mixture on affected area once a day until the skin disorder is cured.

Here is another remedy for cure Psoriasis. Take 30 grams of fresh chives cut to ½ inch long and take 30 grams of garlic pilled together put in a blender to make the paste. Use a microwave warm up the paste and rub the paste on affected skin once a day for a week. Psoriasis could be cured, if not completely cured continue to use the remedy.

Remedy for Shingles

In an ancient Chinese herbal medicine book it is said bees wax has therapeutic effects of cleansing toxic heat, relieve pain, and healing skin ulcer. I was told this remedy can stop pain immediately and if use it to treat shingles, the shingles can be cured with one treatment.

Heat the bees wax to melt, apply the melted bees wax on the affected skin 3 to 4 mm thick. The pain will stop immediately. The problem is the bees wax melting temperature is 70 degree that can cause burn to the skin.

The temperature too low will affect the efficacy. To avoid this problem in Chinese medicine practice we put the bees wax on the skin at a low temperature then use moxibustion therapy to warm up the bees wax. If you want to try this remedy you can use a cigarette to warm up the wax.

Remedy for Dermatitis, Eczema, and Ringworm

To treat skin disorders, such as Dermatitis, Eczema, and Ringworm commonly used remedies are steroid creams and ointments. These remedies contain hormones. Long-term using them can lead to large pores, telangiectasia, and accelerate skin aging. Try the following natural remedy without side effects.

Cut a slice of white turnip and dip turnip into vinegar, then use the turnip rub on affect skin for three minutes. Use this remedy three times a day for a week can cure some skin disorder.

Remedy for Vaginal Itching or Anus Itching

Vaginal itching in most cases is caused by vaginal yeast infection. Many women taking antibiotic to stop itching but only can get temperate relief. Vaginal yeast infection related to lack of estrogen. Drink soybean milk can help improving the condition. This natural remedy can help stop the itching.

Pour 500ml of vinegar in a cooking pot and add 5 grams of salt in the vinegar. Warm up the vinegar over low heat. Use the vinegar wash vagina 3 times a day until the symptom is gone.

To treat Vaginitis, at night before go to sleep put three vitamin C pills in vagina and keep doing it for a week.

Remedies for Diabetes

Remedy for Diabetes (1)

We eat okras as vegetable. Okra originally came from Africa. Its seedling, leaves, flower, and fruit all are edible. Oil extracted from okra's seeds can be used for cooking and therapeutic use. Okra has amazing healing effect. It is rich in vitamin A, B, C, and trace elements like iron, potassium, and calcium. Okra contains 15%-26% protein that can protect gastric wall mucus to prevent stomach cancer and colon cancer. It is also beneficial to liver, intestines, and skin. For therapeutic use it can be used to treat diabetes, Gastritis, stomach ulcer, Hemorrhoids, edema, and urinary tract infection. If your blood glucose is high you can try this natural remedy to lower your blood sugar lever. Some diabetic patients had insulin injection for years they use this remedy replaced insulin injection.

Take two fresh okra pods cut off both end and slice lengthwise. Soak the okras in a glass of drinking water. Cover the glass and leave it in room temperature overnight.

114

The next morning remove the okra and drink the water. Keep drinking okra soaked water every day for two weeks the blood glucose level can drop to normal range. Some people have already using this simple remedy replaced insulin injection for many years.

Remedy for Diabetes (2)

Ingredients: 1000 grams soybeans washed clean, 500g fresh ginger cut to thin slices, four bottles of rice vinegar, a large glass jar

First put a layer of soybeans in the glass jar, on the soybeans put a layer of ginger, then a layer of soybeans cover the ginger and a layer of ginger cover the soybeans until put all the soybeans and the ginger in the jar. Pour vinegar into the jar until the vinegar covered the soybeans and the ginger. Seal the jar for 4 months. After 4 months, every day eat 10 to 20 soybeans and 2 to 3 slices of ginger after dinner for one week. Check the blood glucose the result should show the improvement. Keep using this remedy for three months blood glucose level should be normal and the condition will be stable.

Remedy for Diabetes (3)

This remedy can balance blood glucose, boost energy, and relieve the dryness.

Ingredients: ½ lemon peeled, 250 grams of raw pumpkin peeled and have pumpkin seeds removed

Cut pumpkin into small pieces. Put pumpkin and lemon together in a blender and add a little water, blend the ingredients to make smoothies. Take the smoothies twice a day and each time take half amount of the smoothies. Keep using this remedy for a week should have significant result. Keep using this remedy until the blood glucose reading is normal and stable.

More Remedies for Self Cure

Remedy for Improve General Health

This remedy is very popular in Japan because of its therapeutic effects on many health issues. Use this remedy can promote blood circulation, balance blood pressure, lower blood glucose. It is very beneficial to brain and eyes. Use it regularly can prevent and improve Alzheimer's disease, Cataract, Presbyopia, blurred vision, and eye fatigue. When I was working on this book my eyes got so tired, sometimes during the night I felt the pain of my eyes. I started to use this remedy until I finished this book. It does make my eyes feel better also keep me very focused on my work. It is said keep using this remedy for a while can read book without reading glasses. Plus by using this remedy can stop frequent urination during the night. One ingredient in this remedy is red wine. Red wine has anti-aging and antioxidants effects, drink small amount of red wine often can help prevent cardiovascular diseases.

Take two medium sized onions peel the brown skin and from the center of the onion cut into 8 equal parts. Place the onion in a glass jar and add 500ml red wine, or use 3 onions with one bottle red wine. Close the jar and store it in a cool place. After a week it is ready to use. Drink 50ml of red wine and eat two pieces of onion every day. Elderly people can drink twice a day, each time drink 20ml of the red wine.

Remedy for Bone Spur

Bone spur usually seen in elderly people. In western medicine study the cause of the bone spur is not clear and there is no treatment available. One day I had to do a house call. A woman at her fifties had bone spur for several months when the pain became unbearable both of her feet couldn't touch the floor. She rushed to a hospital and stayed in the hospital for a week. She didn't receive any treatment then she was told she should go home. According to the theory of Chinese medicine bone spur is related to the dysfunction of kidney. With Chinese herbal remedy and treatment bone spur can be cured with a few treatment sessions. You can try this remedy to take care of this problem yourself.

Cut 50 grams of the fresh ginger to small pieces and put into a blender. Add 2 tablespoons of vinegar and blend the ginger to make paste. At night before go to sleep apply the paste to troubled area, cover it with gauge first and wrap the foot with plastic wrap to stable the gauge. Sleep with it and take it off in the morning. Continue this treatment every day for seven to ten days depend on the condition.

To treat heel pain also can try this remedy. Cut a few slices of turnip skin and cook in boiling water for one minute. Apply the turnip skin on the painful heel when the skin is very warm. Reheat the cool skin and keep apply very warm skin on the heel for 30 minutes. Use this remedy every day for 10 days.

Remedy for Hepatitis B

To use this remedy to cure Hepatitis B you need find one ingredient. This ingredient is free if you can find a eggplant farm, collect some root of eggplant. If use dried eggplant root take 200-300 grams of the ingredient, if use fresh eggplant root take 500 grams of the ingredient, because fresh root is heavier than dried root. Wash them clean and cook them in 500ml of boiling water for 20 minutes. Drain the decoction and set aside. Add 500ml of water in same ingredient cook it again for 20 minutes. Remove the ingredient and mix the decoctions together. Drink one time the decoction per day and each time drink half portion of the decoction. The decoction you made is for two days supply. Then stop taking the decoction for two days. On the fifth day make new decoction for another two days. After taking the decoction for two days and without drinking decoction for two days for total 80 days; that mean you cooked 20 times of the decoction; then you can go to get a blood test the liver condition should be normal. You may drink the decoction once a month for ten month to prevent relapse.

Coarse Salt Remedy for Relieve Pain

This remedy can cure Rheumatoid arthritis, uterine fibroids, lower back pain, Osteoporosis, stomach pain, vomiting, and more. How this remedy can treat so many problems? Because this remedy can be used to treat local problems like arthritis or knee pain, it also can be used to open meridians all over the body. According to Chinese medicine theory if all meridians in a person's body without blockage this person is in perfect health.

This remedy is for external use. Use a piece of fabric to make a bag or a sock can do the same work.

Ingredients: 5LBs of Coarse salt. Coarse salt is unrefined salt look like small rocks. At Chinese supermarkets you still can find them. A large piece of ginger cut to slices. 6 green onions only use white part with the roots cut to 1 inch long.

Place the Coarse salt in a large sauce pan bake and stir over medium heat about 10 minutes. When the salt pops add in ginger and green onions and stir for another 2 minutes. Put all ingredients in the bag and tied the opening. If use microwave put all ingredients in the bag and put the bag in the microwave heat for 5 minutes.

To treat arthritis, lower back pain, or pain in certain area just use salt bag perform fomentation at the local area, keep moving the bag to avoid burn the skin.

To open the meridians let the patient lie on his stomach, start from back of the ankles little by little moving upward, passing the legs, the hips, the lower back, and then following the spine move up until to the neck. Next step is turning the patient over lie on his back. Put the bag on lower abdomen slowly moving up to the stomach area. This treatment is very beneficial to the people with low energy and low body temperature. For people with heat body constitution only use this treatment on local area.

Remedy for Fatty Tumor

It is hard for me to believe banana peel can make tumor disappear or cure skin problem like Psoriasis. When I share this remedy with some people who have fatty tumors no one person care to try it, they prefer to get the "real treatment" to make their tumors disappear. I have treated patients with ovary tumor, uterus tumor, and the tumor on the neck with the massage combine with other therapies. One female patient had a tumor on her neck and her surgery was scheduled in two weeks. After the first session the following week she came to show me her tumor was disappeared completely. Another female patient had an ovary tumor size like a tennis ball she had made an appointment to remove it with surgery. Before the surgery

I treated her tumor with two sessions and the tumor was gone completely after the second session. According to my experience when the fatty tumor is soft with 1 or 2 treatment sessions it will be gone completely, because fatty tumor is the accumulation of fat tissue or mucus, once the circulation improved the tumor will be gone. If it became hard it has to be removed by the surgery. If the fatty tumor doesn't keep growing you don't have to do anything about it. I include this remedy in this book if anyone can try it and get the result like what I was told that will be great.

A middle-aged Chinese man had a tumor on his head and the tumor is hard. His doctor recommended having a surgery to remove it, the cost of the surgery is 5000 Chinese yuan ($830). The man couldn't afford it. A friend told him use banana peel to rub on the tumor. He tried. The next day the tumor ruptured and a lot of pus came out. He cleaned the pus with alcohol and several days later the wound healed itself. It must use ripe banana peel in order to get the good result.

Another man said he had Psoriasis for 30 years. After he using banana peel rub on affected the skin for two months, his Psoriasis was cured. Also I was told banana peel can be used to treat inflammation and stop pain. Smash banana peel to make paste and mix with some ginger juice, apply the paste on the affected area.

It is said the banana peel also can be used to treat hypertension. Each time use 30 grams of dried banana peel to make hot tea. Drink three times per day for one month will see the improvement. Continue to drink banana peel tea for one or two months to make the condition stable.

Remedy for Motion Sickness

Add a little vinegar in a glass of warm water. Before riding a car or a boat drink that glass of water can prevent motion sickness.

Or before riding a car or a boat put a slice of ginger on the belly button and use a bandage to stable it.

Remedy for Dissolve Stones

The peel of Pomegranate is listed in Chinese Herbal medicine as an herb. Its therapeutic functions include treat chronic diarrhea, enhance the function of kidney to treat spermatorrhea and premature ejaculation. For women it can be used to treat uterine bleeding and vaginal discharge that is due to kidney instability.

Pomegranate can dissolve the stones in the body. This remedy can be used to eliminate gallbladder stones and kidney stones. Wash a Pomegranate clean and with the skin cut to several pieces. Put the Pomegranate in a cooking pot and add one gallon of water. Cook the Pomegranate in boiling water until the water turned to red.

Drink the pomegranate decoction as many times as you can. Same Pomegranate can cook 2 to 3 times.

Remedy for Eliminating Stones from body

Ingredients: One cucumber peeled and chopped, cut a celery from the middle, you will use half of the celery that connect to root, wash it clean and chopped, one lemon peeled and cut, ¼ cup of pine nuts or cashew nuts.

Put all ingredients in a blender and make the paste. After take the paste out of the blender add one tablespoon of honey and stir it even. Eat the paste once a day during 5pm to 6pm can eliminate all stones from body.

Remedy for Bone Fracture

Bone fracture is very painful and need take three months to heal. For elderly people will need longer time to heal. For serious bone fracture you need rush to a hospital let a doctor place a cast to stable the fractured bone. After the cast is removed you can use this remedy to promote healing. For mild bone fracture you can use this remedy right way. This remedy can treat bone fracture, wound, carbuncles, sore, and skin ulcer. Soak 25 grams of dried black fungus in warm water for 2 hours. Put socked black fungus and two tablespoons of dark brown sugar in a blender to make paste. Apply the black fungus paste on injured area and use gauze wrap it. Change the paste once a day. The healing result is amazing.

Remedy for Leg Cramps

It is said 70% of people at age over 50 have experienced leg cramps during the night. After the cramps released the tenderness can still last for a while. There are some factors that can cause leg cramps, such as dehydrated, diabetes, Parkinson disease, Anemia, low blood glucose, and endocrine disorders. In an ancient Chinese medicine book it said leg cramps are related to the disorder of liver and sugar can ease the cramps.

Add one teaspoon brown sugar in a cup of hot water, drink it before go to bed. Drink one time the brown sugar decoction can stop cramps for 1 to 2 weeks.

Remedy for Boost Energy and Replenish Blood

Some people's hands and feet are always cold even they live in hot environment that is one of the symptoms of energy and blood deficiency. Use this remedy often can improve the physical constitution. Place 5 dried Chinese dates, 5 dried Longan, and 3 slices of ginger together in a cooking pot, add 2 cups of water and cook the ingredients in boiling water for 15 minutes. After turn off the heat add one teaspoon dark brown sugar in the decoction and drink it as hot tea.

A Natural Therapy for Cure Stroke and Bell's Palsy without Sequela

To treat stroke take 500 grams of fresh ginger root finely chopped put in a bowl and add half bottle of drinking alcohol in the bowl. Place the bowl in a steamer steam for 15 minutes. Wrap the ginger in a piece of cloth and tied it up. The therapist holds wrapped ginger and press along the patient's spine up and down for 30 minutes. After the treatment let the patient drinks some hot ginger decoction. During the treatment the patient must avoid to eat sugar and meat until the stroke is completely cured.

Bell's palsy is paralysis on one side of a person's face. The cause of Bell's palsy is unknown to western medical study and there is no reliable treatment available. If the patient received glucose drip treatment the condition will become very difficult to recover. With Chinese medicine treatment and take Chinese herbal remedy can help make quick recovery. For self cure the patient can treat himself by using the same way to make ginger wrap and hold it press on the whole face. Finish the treatment drink some hot ginger decoction. Use this therapy once a day until the symptoms completely gone.

Chapter Four

Remedies for Gynecological and Pediatric Disorders

Remedy for Painless Childbirth

In my practice the last couple of years the number of pregnant women looking for induced labor treatment has increased. In Chinese medicine the natural way to induce labor is massage therapy, acupuncture, and herbal remedies. For most women giving birth to a child is not an easy task. When I gave birth to my son I almost lost my own life. This remedy can make the labor process become easy and painless.

This remedy only needs one ingredient and it is free. In each walnut there is a thin slice of wood between the walnut meats. In Chinese herbal medicine it is called Fen Xin Mu. I don't know if there is an English name for it since nobody pays attention to it but this small piece of wood has amazing healing effects. Cook 5 grams of Fen Xin Mu in boiling water for 20 minutes. Pregnant women from the 36th week can start drinking Fen Xin Mu decoction until the due date. When the contractions start drink 2 cups of Fen Xin Mu decoction. It is said the mom can relax and take a nap. After the nap she is ready for the baby come into this world.

Besides inducing labor Fen Xin Mu is very beneficial to the kidneys. Use 3 grams of Fen Xin Mu to make the decoction. Drink one cup of the decoction in the morning and one cup in the evening to treat frequent urination, urgent urination, impotence, and other sexual dysfunction symptoms. Elderly people can keep using this remedy to relieve lower back pain and strengthen weak knees, and improve hearing. This herb is very effective in treating chronic insomnia. Drink one cup of the decoction an hour before going to the bed. This herb will not cause any side effects and everyone can use this remedy for good health.

By the way, I have advice for breast feeding women. When you are angry do not feed your babies because your milk could cause your babies diarrhea. If you are very anger your milk is toxic. This is confirmed by scientific experiment.

Remedies for Infertility

For infertile men and women folic acid is a very important supplement. Men with low sperm content may be caused by lack of folic acid. Folic acid is one kind of vitamin that helps with the synthesis of DNA and conducive to infant neurological development. Unpolished grains contain plenty of Folic acid. To treat male infertility can eat 15g Gou Qi berries every evening, keep eating Gou Qi berries for a few months, and meanwhile reduce sexual activity.

For women infertility if it is due to irregular menstruation. There are many factors that could cause irregular menstruation, such as heat or cold accumulation in uterus, blood deficiency, emotional disturbances, and indulgence in sexual life, etc. The treatment and herbal remedies of Chinese medicine are very effective in treating gynecological disorders for both men and women.

Women can use this food remedy to increase their chance of getting pregnant. Take 50 grams of threaded fresh ginger, two tablespoons of sesame seeds, and 2 tablespoons of brown sugar, mix all the ingredients in a saucepan and bake over low heat until the brown sugar melts to make a pan cake. Eat the cake as a snack. Keep using this remedy for 2 to 3 months.

Or take 250 grams of white turnip and 50 grams of fresh ginger. Cut the both ingredients in slices and cook them in boiling water for 15 minutes. Turn off the heat and add one tablespoon of brown sugar. Drink the decoction from the first day of menstruation to the last day of menstruation.

Remedy for Painful Menstruation

A lot of women have the experience of painful menstrual cramps during the first two days of their period. Western medical studies believe menstrual cramps caused by hormonal imbalance leads to uterine contractions. According to Chinese medicine painful menstruation is due to the unbalanced emotions or blood stagnation in the uterus. This simple remedy can eliminate blood stagnation and stop the cramps.

Ingredients: 15 grams of dried Shan Zha (Hwathorn), five slices of fresh ginger, one tablespoon of dark brown sugar

First cook the ginger and the Shan Zha in boiling water for five minutes. Remove the ginger and the Shan Zha from the decoction. Add one teaspoon of dark brown sugar in the decoction and drink it as hot tea.

Use this remedy 2 to 3 times a day during the first couple of days of menstruation to avoid painful cramps, eliminate blood clots, and prevent uterine fibroids. Drinking hot ginger tea also can stop various types of hemorrhage especially chronic uterine bleeding.

A Simple Treatment for Painful Menstruation

The procedure of treating painful menstruation: Take 1/3 of cotton from a regular cotton ball to make a small cotton ball. Dip the small cotton ball in 75% alcohol and place the small cotton ball in the patient's external auditory meatus. After several hours the small cotton ball will be self discharged. If not, take it out the next day. You may only put one cotton ball in one ear or put a cotton ball in both ears. If the patient is suffering dysmenorrhea with headache or dizziness, for left side headache put the cotton ball in the right ear; for right side headache put the cotton ball in the left ear.

Attention: Move slowly! When putting the cotton ball into the patient's ear move slowly to avoid touching the eardrum and causing dizziness. Because the alcohol is cold, hold the cotton ball in the external ear canal for several seconds then put it in slowly.

After placing the cotton ball in the ear most people will get pain relief in several minutes. Over 90% of patients will feel the pain stop in 30 minutes. This remedy is used for immediate relief but it doesn't treat the cause of dysmenorrhea.

Remedy for Morning Sickness

Morning sickness is a commonly seen disorder appearing in early stages of pregnancy. According to Chinese medicine theory the cause of this problem is due to weakness of the stomach Qi (energy). The nature of stomach Qi is moving downward, with strong stomach Qi food is pushed downward for the next step of metabolism. A pregnant woman with weak stomach Qi will have a feeling of food stuck in the stomach or moving up. For a mild condition keep a slice of ginger in the mouth or drink hot ginger tea in the morning to ease morning sickness. For a more serious condition squeeze 50ml of chive juice and 10ml of ginger juice and mix them together. Add a little brown sugar and heat up, drinking the juice before breakfast.

Remedy for Menopausal Syndrome

Most women at around age 50 will experience some symptoms of menopausal syndrome, such as hot flashes, night sweats, easily becoming emotional like sadness and irritability, blood pressure imbalance, gaining weight, and depression. According to the theory of Chinese medicine menopausal Syndrome is due to kidney yin deficiency. Acupuncture treatment and Chinese herbal remedies can treat menopausal syndrome very effectively. Without proper treatment menopausal syndrome can last more than ten years. I was told that using this remedy for 15 days can improve symptoms significantly.

Ingredients: 150 grams of honey, 120 grams of Bai He (dried Lily bulb) powder

Mix the two ingredients well and put in a steamer and steam for one hour. After the temperature cools down, eat half of the remedy in the morning and the other half in the evening. This is for one day's use. You can increase the amount of the ingredients to make the remedy enough for several days' use.

Remedy for Children with Chronic Bronchitis

Chronic bronchitis is one of the commonly seen pediatric diseases. Children with chronic bronchitis suffer productive cough which is worse during the night. By using this remedy for 3 to 6 months chronic bronchitis can be cured, and using this remedy also can prevent children from catching cold.

Ingredients: One bottle of rice vinegar, 500 grams of rock sugar

Soak the rock sugar in rice vinegar for 5 days, and shake it evenly. Every day before breakfast take 15ml of the vinegar and in the evening before going to bed take 15ml of the vinegar. There are no side effects and the taste is easy for children to accept.

Remedy for Fever and Cough

Some children very easily to get fever and cough due to their weak physical constitution. Using antipyretics can damage children's immune system. This remedy can bring down a fever quickly without any side effects. Other benefits of this remedy include curing mouth ulcers and stopping cough.

Take a heart of Chinese cabbage chopped (all yellow leaves can be used). Soak half cup of soybeans in cold water for one hour. Cook soaked soybeans in boiling water for 40 minutes first, then add the Chinese cabbage. Cook for 5 minutes more. Drink the decoction when it is warm.

Why some children at the age of 1 to 5 are restless during the night and always easily cry and are fretful during the day? This is caused by parents feed them refined foods, fatty foods, chocolate, and sweets. These high-calorie foods lead to internal heat and the kids have no way to vent. Use millet to make porridge. Feed the children with the porridge can clear internal heat and calm down the irritation.

Remedy for Infantile Diarrhea

Infantile diarrhea is a commonly seen problem in pediatrics. To prevent this problem make sure the baby's abdomen is always covered when the baby is sleeping and avoid feeding the baby cold food or overfeeding. If your baby has diarrhea you can feed the baby the following congee as a meal. Put 2 tablespoons of rice in a saucepan and bake over low heat until the rice turns light yellow. Grind the rice into powder and put the rice powder in a pot. Add some water and cook for 2 minutes. It will become light congee. Turn off the heat and add a little dark brown sugar. Feed the baby with the congee to stop the diarrhea immediately.

Remedy for Infantile Spitting up Milk

Here is a tip for a mom with a new born baby. Because a new born baby's digestive system is not developed well enough to handle what they eat, two problems often seen in new born babies are spitting up milk and diarrhea. To solve these two problems the mom can feed her baby with a little warm, light ginger tea before feeding the baby milk.

Chapter Five

Remedies for Hypertension

Hypertension is a western medical term for high blood pressure. In the first four chapters you already found some remedies that can be used to treat Hypertension. The reason I use one chapter to talk about Hypertension is because Hypertension is one of the most popular health problems and the medications being used to control high blood pressure can lead to many other chronic diseases, such as diabetes, obesity, depression, liver disease, kidney disease, heart disease, and even cancer. Most people around the age of 50 are diagnosed with hypertension and start taking prescription drugs for the rest of their lives. As time pass they will develop other diseases and take more prescription drugs until they die of one of those diseases. How can those diseases develop by using antihypertensive drugs?

Antihypertensive drugs have side effects on the liver. Many hypertension patients have a big bloated abdomen that indicates a disorder of the liver and in the digestive system.

135

One of the functions of the liver is to remove toxins in the blood. When liver detoxification function decreases hypertension patients develop high cholesterol and cardiovascular diseases.

The side effects of Antihypertensive drugs can cause disorder in the digestive system. The organs involved are stomach, spleen, and the gallbladder. Digestion disorder can cause acid reflux and abdominal bloating. Dysfunction of the digestive system makes the metabolic process difficult. Spleen is a very important organ for metabolism. It is responsible for transforming nutrients to energy and blood. Malfunction of the spleen will lead to low energy, upper body edema, and gaining weight. Almost all antihypertensive drugs are diuretics that have side effects on the function of the kidneys. Dysfunction of the kidneys can cause edema in the lower extremities and sexual disorders.

Antihypertensive drugs are acidic. Long-term use of high blood pressure medication can make the patient's physical constitution become acidic. Almost all cancer patients' physical constitution is acidic.

I would like to reveal the truth of hypertension. **Humans are creators. Mankind has created a fantastic material world and at the same time we also created human diseases. Hypertension and the medication being used to treat this disease were created after someone invented**

the blood pressure meter, and set up a normal blood pressure reading of 120/80. Hypertension is a human creation. With blood pressure meters doctors can monitor the patient's blood pressure. If your blood pressure reading is higher than the normal reading you will be diagnosed with having the disease of hypertension and your doctor will prescribe drugs for you to control your blood pressure. Most likely you will take those drugs for the rest of your life. Western medical practice focuses on the reading of the blood pressure and how to control the number. In fact high blood pressure is a symptom not a disease. Blood pressure meters brain washed people by their doctors and health care professionals. They were told if they don't take high blood pressure medication they could die of heart attack and stroke. By taking antihypertensive drugs can you really prevent heart attack and stroke? My father took antihypertensive drugs for more than 20 years and died of a heart attack. Antihypertensive drugs are acidic and can damage the blood vessel walls causing blood vessel rupture leading to stroke or heart attack. Blood pressure meters and antihypertensive drugs do not make people healthier. The side effects of the drugs can cause more health problems. This is why so many men and women after age 50 will develop multiple diseases such as high cholesterol, diabetes, heart disease, arthritis, and cancer? In my practice very often I hear people say "I am a big mess." I feel so sorry for these people who have no idea how they messed up their health. They don't know without a doctor's help it is not easy to mess up their bodies. Most cases are started from taking medication for high blood pressure.

In Traditional Chinese Medicine there is no such disease called Hypertension but the treatment and herbal remedies in Chinese medicine can treat this symptom very effectively. In Chinese medicine practice high blood pressure is not considered a difficult case. My own practice records show Hypertension patients can quit medication easily with a few sessions of treatment and a few bottles of Chinese herbal remedies. Chinese herbal remedies are intended to balance and strengthen the body's own systems, so that eventually the patient can stop taking the herbal remedies and not become dependent on them. The following are real cases that show how easy it is to quit antihypertensive drugs.

Case 1: A 64-year-old male patient wanted to quit high blood pressure medication because he realized the medication he was taking caused him to gain weight and become impotent. His health condition made him feel very stressful at work and in his relationship. According to the information I got and Chinese medicine diagnostic methods I think he is a very healthy man, his problem is due to the side effect of the medication and unbalanced emotion that causes toxic heat accumulation in his liver. With one treatment session and two bottles of herbal remedies his blood pressure went back to normal. After two years he is still doing very well without taking any medication.

Case 2: A 71-year-old male patient had been taking high blood pressure medication for more than 20 years. At his first visit he was overweight with a big stomach. He complains he has very low energy, poor digestion, acid reflux, kidney stones, lower back pain, swollen legs and ankles. He has been taking medications for high blood pressure, high cholesterol, and one medication for heart artery blockage that he had to stop taking because of the serious side effects. In short his condition is a mess.

The treatment plan for him is using the therapies in Chinese medicine to boost his energy, enhance the function of his kidneys and his heart. He took two herbal remedies but none of them is for lower blood pressure. One is to improve the function of his heart and promote the blood circulation of the heart. Another remedy is to enhance the function of his kidneys. Plus I asked him to stop drinking cold drinks. Two weeks later on his third visit he told me he felt his heart is fine and his energy is much better. He went to see his doctor two days ago because he felt dizziness and found out his blood pressure reading was 110/65. His doctor let him stop taking high blood pressure medication. He lost some weight, no more swelling on his legs and ankles. He started working out, and acid reflux was improved just by changing his habit of drinking cold water. How can he quit the medication in such short time? The treatment approach of Chinese medicine focuses on treating the cause, improving the function of the organic systems not the blood pressure reading.

Case 3: A 57-year-old female patient had been taken high blood pressure medication for more than 5 years. On her first visit she complained that suddenly she started vomiting and had diarrhea with abdominal pain and cramps. I treated her as digestion disorder. On her second visit she told me the vomiting and the diarrhea were caused by the side effects of a new high blood pressure medication she was taking. Her doctor let her try a new blood pressure medication. During the first two months she didn't have any bad reaction, so when she started having vomiting and diarrhea she didn't realize that it was the side effects of the new medication. The treatment I did for her didn't stop the vomiting and the diarrhea until the health insurance stopped paying for the new medication because it was too expensive. When she was fighting with the insurance company she ran out of her medication. Without the medication her vomiting and diarrhea stopped. She had a few sessions of the treatment and took one herbal remedy called "Liu Wei Di Huang Wan" that she found very helpful for improving her health condition. This herbal remedy is not particularly for lowering blood pressure, it is a very popular remedy being used among the Chinese people who are over 45 because this remedy has the benefits of replenishing the essence of liver and kidney. For most people after reaching age 45 the kidney's metabolism slows down leading to liver and kidney essence deficiency and cause blood pressure to go up. To this day this patient quit her medication for more than one year.

In today's health market full of therapies and drugs, they are new and expensive. My advice is you can pursue new styles of fashion, car or cell phone but do not try new medicine. Regarding medicine the older remedies are safer. I am sure no one wants to be a laboratory rat.

Remedy for Resistant Hypertension

A retired chief physician in China shared this remedy and his experience. At age 70 he already had hypertension for more than 10 years. Even taking Western prescription medication his blood pressure reading is always at 180/110. After using this food remedy his blood pressure reading stayed at 130/80. He felt his energy is better. What really surprised him is that his Osteoporosis and blurred vision improved, his cardiac hypertrophy and irregular heartbeats are getting better. Even his gray hair turned darker.

Take one cup of black beans and wash them clean. Use a saucepan to bake the beans over medium heat for 5 minutes. Then turn to low heat and bake for another 5 minutes. Turn off the heat and wait for the beans cool down. Put the black beans in a glass jar and add in rice vinegar until the vinegar covers the beans. Store the jar in a refrigerator for ten days. After 10 days eat 7 to 10 beans and drink one tablespoon of the vinegar every day to balance blood pressure, reduce LDL cholesterol, and prevent Arteriosclerosis.

Remedy for High Blood Pressure

Ingredients: 250 grams of rock sugar, 250 ml of vinegar

Put the rock sugar and the vinegar in a cooking pot. Cook over low heat until the rock sugar melts. Turn off the heat and wait for the decoction cool down, store the decoction in a container. Drink the decoction three times a day after each meal. Each time take 2 tablespoons of the decoction. After taking the decoction 3 to 4 days check your blood pressure. If the blood pressure decreases to the normal reading you may start reducing your prescription medication from taking the medication every day to taking it every other day. Keep using the remedy for another week. If your blood pressure is lower than the normal reading you need stop taking your medication. Continue taking the remedy for another two weeks without medication. If your blood pressure reading is normal and stable you can stop using this remedy.

Remedy for High Blood Pressure

Heat up one gallon of water and add 2 tablespoons of baking soda in the water. Use the baking soda water soaking the feet for 20 minutes every day for one week.

A 70-year-old man had high blood pressure for 20 years. His blood pressure reading was 180/90. Using baking soda decoction to soak his feet for one week his blood pressure has been normal for two years.

Another simple remedy for Hypertension is using 100-150 grams of fresh celery. Squeeze the juice and add a little honey to it. Drink the celery juice once a day to keep normal blood pressure.

Remedy for High Blood Pressure

Peanut is a very popular food. We eat peanuts and peanut butter but most people don't know the whole plant has therapeutic value. The red skin of the peanut can replenish blood. The shell of peanut can be used to treat insomnia. If you live close to a peanut farm collect some peanut plants wash them clean and leave them at a place with good ventilation to let them dry.

50 grams of dried peanut plant (bar and leaves), if you use fresh peanut plant you will need 150 grams of the ingredient. Wash them clean and cut the peanut plant to small pieces. Cook the ingredient in a half gallon of boiling water for 15 minutes. Remove the ingredient and drink the decoction as hot tea. Drink this decoction every day until

the blood pressure reading is normal and stable. This remedy also has the effect of cleansing toxic heat in the blood and lowering cholesterol.

Chapter Six

Food Remedies for Cancer

Cancer is a curable and preventable disease. There are many ways to prevent and cure cancer but people are not aware of them. Very often I hear people say fighting cancer but the reality is that in most fighting cancer cases the lives are lost in fighting cancer battles. Medical research has not fully understood the cause of cancer and the treatment methods are as harmful as cancer itself. To fight cancer chemotherapy and radiation therapy are used to kill cancer cells but at the same time these therapies also kill the normal cells as well. Many cancer patients are not dead from the cancer but from the harsh treatment. Among those cancer survivors many people will suffer the side effects of the cancer treatment for the rest of their lives. In this chapter you shall find the remedies to prevent cancers and the remedies to cure cancers. Regarding how to prevent cancer I felt speechless when I watched the news that Angelina Jolie had double mastectomy surgery done to prevent breast cancer and she also had her ovaries removed to prevent ovarian cancer. Angelina Jolie is an actress, she didn't study medicine but her doctor doesn't seem to know better than her. A lot of women are already suffering the side effects of removal of the uterus and ovaries. Every organ plays an important role in the whole body system and each organ does not independently exist. The organs in the whole organic system are connected and rely on each other to function. Cancer cells could develop in any tissue, therefore, by removing organs to prevent cancers is a very shallow and ignorant approach. According to Chinese medicine theory cancer is not a genetic disease same as high blood pressure, diabetes, and many other chronic diseases. My mother and one of my sisters had breast cancer but trace back several generations there was no one person who had cancer in our family. This is true in all other cancer patients' families, because only 40 years ago cancer was not a commonly seen disease. What triggered a normal cell to become cancerous has not been understood by medical studies yet. At cancer hospitals in China I noticed besides food remedies are shared by cancer patients, also there are some people distribute healing mantras. They said they themselves or their loved ones had cancer and were cured by chanting mantras without receiving any medical treatment. After they were cured they printed and distributed the mantras at cancer hospitals to help others. What is a mantra? Mantras are very ancient knowledge and the science of the future. It is part of the practice in the highest level of Chinese medicine and Buddhist teaching. 2500 years ago Sakyamuni the founder of the Buddhist teaching taught his disciples a mantra to cure cancers. How to use the mantras to cure cancers or any kind of ailments? The most commonly used method is chanting the mantra to charge a glass of water and after the patient drank the water he was cured. Cancer patients can use the mantra to cure themselves. At a cancer hospital in Beijing I met two men who were distributing the mantra and telling people their own stories.

One man said he came to this hospital for a nose bleeding problem and was diagnosed with Nasopharyngeal Carcinoma. He was so scared and before he left the hospital someone gave him a flier. On the flier was printed the mantra and the explanation of how to use it. From that day he chanted the mantra 21 times in the morning and 21 times in the evening, soon the tumor on his neck disappeared and his nose bleeding stopped. He was cured. He was so grateful that sometimes he would print the mantra and distribute it at cancer hospitals.

Another man's story is that he was diagnosed as having stomach cancer. While he was staying in a cancer hospital waiting for his family borrowing money from relatives and friends to pay for his surgery he got a flier with the mantra to cure cancer. He followed the instruction, every day he placed a cup of water in front of a Buddha's picture and chanted the mantra 108 times, after chanting the mantra he drunk the water. Since he started chanting the mantra he had three bowel movements every day. Less than a month later his test results showed the tumor was gone. He printed 1000 fliers to send out at the cancer hospital helping other cancer patients.

I had done some research and believe the deepest cause of cancer is far beyond the category of physical. I hope in the near future I can share the information with whoever wants to know. After you read this chapter you will realize that the cancer prevention and cure are much easier than you thought.

So far conventional medical practice focuses on cancers and cancer treatment, there is no research done on those people who had cancer and were cured without receiving any medical treatment. Here are some causes that could lead to cancer patients being cured without medical treatment.

1. Some cancer patients were cured after they had high fever. Cancer cells cannot survive in high temperature. Fever is one of the actions the immune system takes to fight the disease. If your body temperature is slightly higher than the normal body temperature you can be immune to most diseases including cancer. Some people's body temperature is always slightly lower than the normal body temperature this indicates their immune system is weak. What is immunity? Using western medicine theory to explain the immune system is quite complicated. According to Chinese medicine theory good energy, ample

blood, and good circulation are invincible immunity. What is energy? Energy is heat. That is why increases in body temperature can enhance the immunity. Think about this question: What is the difference between a living person and a dead body? A living person has energy. In a dead body there is no energy. A living person's body is warm, a dead body is cold. In my practice I noticed many commonly seen health issues, such as Hypertension, obesity, and depression, etc. are due to low energy and low body temperature. There are many factors that lead to low body temperature, such as lack of exercise, excessively consuming cold food or drinks, and overeating. For people with depression, kidney stones, high blood pressure, and diabetes by using the herbal remedies and the therapies of Chinese medicine to strengthen their energy and increase their body temperature they can quit prescription drugs in a few weeks.

Normal body temperature is about 37 degrees Celsius. Body temperature decreases can lead to a series of reactions. When body temperature drops to 36 degrees the person's ability to respond and make decisions will be weakened. When the body temperature decreases to 35 degrees it will be difficult for the person to write his name and walk. When the body temperature decreases to 33 degrees the person will be completely irrational. When the body temperature decreases to 32 degrees most people will collapse. When the body temperature decreases to 30 degrees many people will lose consciousness. At this point the body already gives up to maintaining body temperature. Breathing reduced to 2 to 3 times per minute. When the body temperature decreases to 28 degrees the person will experience irregular heartbeat. When the body temperature decreases to 20 degrees the body starts to become cold and heartbeat stops but the person is not completely dead yet, because extreme cold can slow down the cells collapse to avoid permanent damage. Then how much is the human body's lowest survival temperature? Theoretically the limit is zero, at this temperature ice begins to form inside the body and all cells will be destroyed.

In recent years people are very conscious about eating healthy. They are educated through lectures, workshops, and magazines to eat organic food, low carbohydrate food, low calorie food, gluten free food, and juicing but the results are not 100% positive. A lot of people with symptoms of low energy and blood deficiency claim they eat very healthy. People should choose food based on their physical constitution. If a person with low energy, cold limbs, edema, and diarrhea eat low calorie food and are juicing the condition can worse. In order to make your body full of vitality you should add those energy foods to your diet. The treatment and the herbal remedies in Chinese medicine are focused on strengthening energy, nourishing blood, and promote circulation. Your own immune system can inhibit cancer cells growth and spread.

2. The second cause of some cancer patients being cured without medical treatment due to disappearance of the factors that lead to cancer. Cancer cells need a toxic environment to grow and cancer cells die in clean blood. A Russian scientific experiment discovered that cancer cells die in a new born baby's blood because a new born baby's blood is toxic free. Science study also discovered that at the old age all people have cancer cells in their bodies but without a toxic environment the cancer cells do not grow and spread. Where do the toxins come from? How to keep our bodies toxin free? In most people's mind the toxins come from the food we eat. Foods are not the main source of the toxins. The major source of toxins is chemical drugs, unbalanced emotions, and the radiations in our environment.

3. Be relaxed and be humble. Personality does have a connection with cancer and women are more easily caught in unbalanced emotions. According to Chinese medicine the emotions of worry and anger can affect the liver, causing liver Qi stagnant. From an acupuncture chart you can see the liver meridians passing through women's breasts and uterus. If liver meridians blocked at the breasts or the uterus are not being treated, over time it could lead to tumors and cancer.

4. A person having cancer if his or her physical constitution changed becoming slightly alkaline the cancer can be cured without medical treatment. 85% of cancer patients' physical constitution is acidic. Healthy people's blood pH is slightly alkaline, about pH 7.35-7.45. If you want to be healthy you need to keep your body pH balanced. PH balance indicates your internal balance of Acid and Alkaline. If your body pH is slightly Acidic you are more easily get sick. If your body pH is slightly alkaline you are healthy and look younger. Maintaining the body in a slightly alkaline constitution is the key in preventing cancer.

How to differentiate an acidic constitution?

- Usually people with acidic constitution are overweight with big abdomen, have stiffness in the neck and the shoulders.
- Very often feel dry in the mouth, odor in the mouth, and prefer cold drinks.
- Very sensitive to hot environment, and easy to get irritated due to stagnation of energy and the accumulation of internal heat.
- Dull and rough skin.
- A little exercise can cause fatigue and gasp for breath.

What are the causes of acidic constitution?

- Excessive intake of acidic food and the food with strong flavor.
- Unhealthy life style, staying up late and bad eating habits, overeating and skipping meals.
- Unbalanced emotions at home or at work, and mental stress.

The following is the pH of common foods.

Foods with strong acidity: egg yolk, cheese, sweet snacks, and many prescription drugs are strong acid agents.

Foods that are acidic: ham, bacon, chicken, pork, beef, bread, butter.

Foods with weak acidity: rice, peanuts, beer, and wine.

Foods that are weak alkaline: red beans, apple, cabbage, Tofu.

Foods that are alkaline: soybeans, carrot, tomato, banana, orange, lemon, vinegar, egg white, straw berries, Spinach, and green vegetables.

Foods that are alkali: grapes, grape wine, green tea, seaweed.

Food Remedy for Uterine Cancer

250 grams of potatoes washed clean, keep the skin, squeeze one cup of potato juice. Drink the raw potato juice

5 times a day and each time drink one cup. While using this remedy the timing is very important. Drink the raw tomato juice at 8:30am, 10:30am, 1:30pm, 4:30pm, and before going to bed drink one cup of the juice.

Instead of using potatoes you can use 250 grams of unripe green papaya. Squeeze the papaya juice and drink the juice with the same timing as using potato.

Remedy for All Kinds of Cancer

Kelp (seaweed) has therapeutic effect of eliminating tumors. Add kelp in cancer patient's diet to enhance immunity and inhibit cancer cell's development.

Soaking 40g dried kelp in cold water overnight and wash it clean. Cook the kelp and 100g of wheat kernels in one gallon of water for 20 minutes. Remove the ingredients and drink the decoction 4 to 5 times per day.

Folk Remedy for Cancer

I was told that this remedy has brought incredible results for a lot of cancer patients. This remedy only needs one ingredient and it is free. When walnuts are picked up from a walnut tree they are covered with a layer of green peel. The dried green walnut peel is what you need. Only dried green walnut peel can be used, do not use the fresh peel. Each time take 250g of dried walnut peel wash clean and soak in one liter cold water for 30 minutes. Cook the walnut peel over high heat until the water is boiling.

Change to low heat and cook for 30 minutes. Remove the walnut peel and drink the decoction as hot tea. Finish the whole decoction in one day, the next day use new ingredients to make new decoction. Use this remedy until cancer is cured. How long for the cancers to be cured? It depends on the patient's condition. So far have successfully cured cases included late stage bone cancer, lung cancer, breast cancer, and late stage liver cancer.

Unpolished Rice Tea Can Stop Cancer Cell development in 3 days

In fact, except the inhibition of cancer cell's development this remedy has the therapeutic effects on several diseases which include break down LDL cholesterol, cleansing the blood, and promoting blood circulation. Its diuretic effect can promote urination. This rice tea is rich in fiber so that it can promote bowel movements to relieve constipation. For different diseases to be cured requires different lengths of time.

*For patients with all kinds of cancer drinking the rice tea for three days can stop the cancer cells development.

*For patients with pancreatic cancer and Jaundice need to keep using this remedy every day for about three months to be cured.

*Patient with Gastric ulcer or duodenal ulcer should drink the rice tea everyday to see improvement in 3 to 10 days.

For complete functional recovery use the remedy for 30 days.

*For patients with Cirrhosis, liver cancer, hypertension, and arthritis keep using the remedy for a year.

*For patients with cataract use the remedy for 4 months to be cured.

Bake 200g of unpolished rice (or brown rice) over low heat until the rice turns light-brown and set aside. Fill one cooking pot with one gallon of water and cook over high heat. When the water is boiling add in baked rice and turn off the heat immediately. Cover the pot and wait for five minutes. Drink the decoction as hot tea.

Attention: Do not drink the rice tea with protein food, for example milk. Do not drink the rice tea with vegetable soup. Do not drink the rice tea with medication. If you need to take Chinese herbal remedy wait for one hour. If you need to take Western medication wait for two hours.

Red Decoction to Reduce Side Effects of Cancer Treatment

This remedy spread in cancer hospitals in China and is used by cancer patients before and during chemotherapy in order to avoid using drugs to increase blood cell count.

All ingredients in this remedy have the therapeutic effect of replenishing blood and increasing blood cell count.

Because all five ingredients are red color people call this remedy red decoction. This remedy is also very beneficial to people with anemia and people with symptoms as dry eyes, dry skin and dry hair.

Ingredients: 10 grams of Chi Xiao Dou (Chinese red beans), 10 grams of Gou Qi berries, 10 grams of Peanuts with the red skin, 8 dried Chinese dates, one tablespoon of dark brown sugar

Put red beans, Gou Qi berries, peanuts, and dates in a cooking pot and add 3 cups of water. Cook for 30 minutes. After the decoction cools down add one tablespoon of dark brown sugar. Drink the decoction once a day.

Remedy for Esophageal Cancer

More than ten years ago a woman in China got esophageal cancer. She was suffering the pain in her chest and felt so helpless. A stranger told her about this remedy. Use a piece of fabric to make a bag. Bake 500 grams of coarse salt in a saucepan until the salt pops. Put hot salt in the bag and tie up the opening. Place the bag on the painful area overnight. She tried. The next day she spit out some blood, the pain was gone and she was cured.

Several years later her sister in law also got esophageal cancer. The hospital let her go home and told her family to prepare a funeral. The woman used the same remedy on her sister-in-law, the next day her sister-in-law spit out some blood, had no more pain in the chest and can eat regular food. Since her sister-in-law was cured eight years passed without recurrence. These people have no medical background and they don't know how this remedy worked. They said what they know is there are no side effects and cost nothing. There are more fantastic natural remedies to cure cancers and other ailments I did not include them in this book because some ingredients in those remedies are herbs. I will share the information in my website if you are interested check: www.naturaltherapywebsite.com.

Chapter Seven

Self-Diagnosis

In order to use food therapy to improve your health, stay healthy, and slow down the aging process, the first step is to pay attention to yourself and the changes of your body. I remember one day my mother looking in the mirror and said "I cannot believe I am so old." My father followed her and said "I cannot believe my daughter is going through menopause." Most of the time we focusing our attention on the world around us until suddenly we fell ill or suddenly we noticed we are old. Those who pay attention to themselves are healthier and look younger. You should develop a self-observation habit. The second step is to recognize the symptoms and make correct self-diagnosis. With the correct diagnosis you can decide which food therapy you are going to use.

People rely on doctors to make diagnose for them. Do you think your doctor knows your body better than yourself? The answer is sometimes they do, most of the time they don't. Your doctor relies on the information you give to him and some test results to make a diagnosis. Sometimes I heard people say "I just had my physical exam done and my doctor said everything is fine but I don't feel fine." Why is this? If your energy is low you don't feel fine but your physical exam doesn't check your energy level. If you have internal heat you will not feel fine but your test doesn't show the internal heat. If cold accumulated in certain areas of your body that could cause pain but your test result doesn't show that. If your body retains water that can cause dizziness and vertigo, you don't feel fine but from you test results your doctor cannot see those disorders. Many out of balance conditions cannot be detected by your physical exam. One day a relative called me and said my 91-year-old nanny has abdominal pain and has spent five days in a hospital and had an overall physical exam, the test results showed she is in perfect health. When I find out her pain is moving, not fixed at one spot, I told the relative take my nanny home and buy one Chinese herbal remedy for her to take. My diagnosis is my nanny's abdominal pain is caused by stagnant gas. Energy and gas are invisible to human eyes. Sometimes the diagnosis only relying on the test result is not enough. It also needs doctor's knowledge and the experience. After my nanny took the Chinese herbal remedy her pain was completely gone the next day.

I would like to share another case with you. A man in his thirties came to see me with severe pain that goes from his lower back to the right side of his groin and radiated down to his right leg. He said he got this pain three days ago and he rushed to the hospital. From x-ray and MRI reports his doctor didn't find anything wrong. After he got home he searched online and found some people sharing their experiences. They said "If you have this kind of pain and you go to western medicine they don't know the cause of the pain. You need to look for someone practicing Chinese medicine. In Chinese medicine they know what is wrong and they know how to treat it." Right away he called me and rushed to my office. According to my experience I knew the pain was caused by hernia. I asked him one question "Did you lift any weight that started this pain?" He said "Yes when I was lifting my girl friend's suitcase I felt this shooting pain." For people with hernia lifting weight can make it worse. Some people without any medical back ground when they heard of this situation they can tell it is hernia by experience. The cause of hernia is energy deficiency. So far there is no technology available to measure a person's energy level and most health issues related to the energy deficiency. In my work I do diagnosis and the treatment at the same time, I always start with massage, by observing the person's skin, touching the muscles, and feel the temperature on certain areas of the body I will get enough information to make a diagnosis. When wild animals get sick they rely on themselves. They know where to find certain herbs to heal themselves. As a human, everyone can learn how to take care of himself and others.

All of us want to be in perfect health but most people are always concerned about diseases rather than their health. In my practice I realized most people have no idea what is healthy. They think having pain in the body is normal because most people have pain. They think dry skin, poor sleep, uncontrolled urination, and looking very old are normal. With this chapter you should get a clear concept of health and always keep yourself in that healthy state. Once you noticed an abnormal condition or felt any discomfort take care of it with your knowledge and food therapy as soon as possible. American people have the spirit of DIY. With Home Depot stores you can take care of your house and save money. With this book you can take care of your health and avoid medical costs. The following check list can help you do self-diagnosis and work on your self-healing.

1. Everyday check how you feel. You should feel energized and have no pain anywhere. Low energy and pain could be the symptoms of early stage of serious disease. Pain could be a warning sign of an internal disorder, do not use painkillers to cover the real problem. For example, stiff neck and shoulder pain are the most commonly seen

complaint in the clinic. In most cases, after taking x-ray the doctors' diagnosis will be herniated disk. Actually some cases of neck and shoulder pain reflect a stressful condition in the heart. The condition may due to heart Qi (energy) deficiency or insufficient blood circulation in the heart. Lower back pain is another commonly seen problem in the clinic. Almost all low back pain cases are diagnosed by doctors as herniated disks. All lower back pain except injury caused pain is related to kidney deficiency. If your kidney is healthy your lower back will be strong. If your kidney energy is weak it can cause vertebrae to press together causing a herniated disk. Physical therapy and chiropractics will not improve your kidney's condition. You can find plenty of food remedies in this book for strengthening energy and essence of the kidney. Even your physical exam didn't show anything wrong you should still use food therapy to boost your energy and treat the pain to prevent the condition from getting worse.

2. Your body should be fit. If you are overweight use food therapy gradually to quit prescription drugs and lose weight. If you have a big belly press it with your hands, if it is soft and with pressure you don't feel pain anywhere your problem is poor metabolism and lack of energy. If your belly is big and hard, and you feel pain or discomfort with the pressure the problem inside is stagnation. Use food remedies to promote metabolism and boost energy or promote circulation.

An overweight person, if he is heavy in upper body and his legs are normal that indicates dysfunction of the digestive system. If his upper body is normal but from waist down is heavy and with lower back pain, swollen of the knees and ankles that indicate the dysfunction of kidneys.

3. Check your sleep. You should fall asleep quickly and deeply. If you experience restless sleep, dry mouth and your tongue is dry as a piece of wood, and also you feel itching in the upper back between scapulas are the signs of your blood glucose is high. High blood glucose not necessarily mean you are diabetic. Reduce the sugar intake especially after dinner to have symptoms improve. Frequent urination during the night is due to kidney deficiency. Drooling during sleep is due to spleen deficiency. Snoring indicates energy deficiency. Profuse sweating during the night is due to Yin deficiency. Eating Gou Qi berries can help to promote Yin energy. Unconsciously clenching the jaw during the day and grinding the teeth during the night is caused by liver blood deficiency. Over sleep indicates very low energy. Usually it is seen in depressed patients. Over sleep can make a person lose more energy. For depression patients exercise is very important for them to overcome the depression. In this book you can find food remedies to improve all these symptoms.

4. You should have a good appetite. With a good appetite you enjoy eating simple, light and a variety of food. People

prefer different foods and flavors. Regarding taste people who are vegetarians and enjoy light flavors are usually intelligent and more sensitive. People who are meat eaters and prefer strong flavors are usually brave and less sensitive. We all know how babies respond the first time they taste a little bit of food, because their bodies are so pure even very light flavors can cause a strong sensation. Preparing food with light flavors is better for health. People who are over the age of 50 should eat a small amount of food for each meal and avoid skipping meals or overeating to protect their appetite. Both skipping meals and overeating can consume stomach and spleen Qi. Have no appetite, stomach bloating and acid reflux after meals are due to the weakness of stomach and spleen Qi (energy).

5. You should have bowel movements once a day and the stool should be firm but not too dry. Some people have many bowel movements a day and they think they have good metabolism. Actually that is the symptom of poor metabolism. If a person's has bowel movements after meals with loose stools and undigested food that indicates very weak metabolism. Early morning diarrhea is related to kidney deficiency. Both conditions should be treated. If you are constipated and the stools are little balls that indicates the liver Qi stagnation. Liver Qi stagnation is caused by unhappy emotions. Elderly people with constipation are usually due to Qi and blood deficiency. Because of Qi deficiency the intestines lack of movement to cause

constipation. Or blood deficiency causes dryness of the intestines lead to constipation.

6. You should urinate 4 to 5 times during the day. Difficult urination, urgent urination, and frequent urination during the day or night are due to dysfunction of the kidneys. Feet are always cold is a symptom of kidney deficiency. Kidney deficiency is a medical term in Chinese medicine. It is not a diagnosis of kidney disease. In Chinese medicine it indicates the dysfunction of the kidneys, or kidney Qi and kidney essence are deficient. With urination problems you don't need to go to see your doctor. In western medicine there is no treatment available. With this book you can take care of urination disorders yourself.

7. A person's complexion can reflect the internal disorders. Pale yellow complexion indicates the person has a digestion disorder that is causing blood deficiency. From a person's complexion you can detect cardiac dysfunctions. Pale complexion indicates cardiac blood insufficiency. Uneven darkness on the face indicates cardiovascular blockage. The whole face darkness indicates kidney deficiency.

8. Your skin should be smooth, not too dry or too wet, and no moles, cysts, nodules, brown spots, and fatty tumors. Nodules grow on the neck and under arm area are caused by accumulated dampness in the body. Drinking seed of Job's tears decoction can eliminate the nodules. Brown

spots on the skin are the symptom of liver blood deficiency. Fatty tumors are caused by stagnant phlegm in the tissue. Dry skin, dry hair, losing hair, and poor memory are the symptoms of blood deficiency. It is not necessary to do a blood test. Food therapy is the best way to keep youth and beauty. Skin rash is due to heat toxins in the blood. Females should have very light hair on the face, arms, and legs. Some women have heavy facial hair that is due to water retention.

9. Symptoms of dry hair, hair loss, dizziness, tinnitus, swollen gums, and teeth getting loose are due to dysfunction of the kidneys.

10. Low energy, poor appetite, stomach bloated even after eating small amounts of food, and feeling sleepy after meals are symptoms of Cirrhosis. Patients with liver diseases like Hepatitis and fatty liver should know for them to be cured food therapy is the best choice, not the prescription drugs. Because once the liver is damaged its function of protein synthesis decreases and lack of protein will lead to Cirrhosis. Therefore Hepatitis patients need to eat **meat soup** for protein supplement. Why eat meat soup? The meat cooked in water for a longer time can defuse biological poison. Once the liver being damaged its detoxification function decreases, therefore the patients should avoid taking too many chemical drugs, including vitamins and supplements. Their diet should have more

vegetables and high protein. They should eat more food with a sour taste like vinegar and avoid pungent flavors.

11. Women with prolonged painful menstruation and heavy bleeding with blood clots, sore back, breast pain, and bloating in pelvic area are symptoms of uterine fibroids. Uterine fibroids should be treated and it is very easy to cure with natural therapies and herbal remedies in Chinese medicine.

By the way many of us had this experience, at lunch time or dinner time we are wondering "What am I going to eat?" Probably you will check your refrigerator to see what you have or just go out to find something to eat. In your mind what you care about is finding something to eat you wouldn't consider the condition of your body. It is already a habit for me to pay attention to the changes of my body and constantly be aware of how I feel. If I feel great or I feel not too well I already have a plan of what I am going to eat for a couple of days. I rarely go out to eat because I eat my meals with purpose that make me interested in preparing meals for myself. Each meal I only need a small amount of food, so that I am very conscious not to put useless food in my stomach. Staying healthy is a life-long thing and it is an everyday thing as well. So make every meal count.

Chapter Eight

Food Therapy for Youth and Beauty

Among all the signs of aging people will pay most attention to the changes of their faces. In order to keep younger looking people can spend a fortune on cosmetic products or even surgery. As a matter of fact the life elixir is produced within our bodies. Anyone who wants to keep younger looking must take good care of the digestive system because that is the power house. Through the digestive system the food is transformed to energy and blood. You must have energy to be alive. What is energy? Energy is life. What is the difference between a living person and a dead body? A dead body is cold and motionless. A living person's body is warm and active. It is energy that warms up the body, pushes the blood to circulate, making the heart beat, enable the brain to think and respond, etc. You must have good energy to reduce the risk of disease, if you are sick you must have energy to overcome disease. For younger looking skin you must have sufficient blood to nourish the skin. Wrinkles, dry skin, pale, and dull skin are due to lack of nourishment.

Here is another Chinese medicine doctor Simiao Sun's story. One day when Dr. Sun was passing a village and saw some villagers carrying a coffin walking toward the cemetery. He noticed there is blood drops from the coffin. He asked the villagers who died. They said a woman died in childbirth. He convince the villagers the woman was not dead yet and asked them to open the coffin. He treated the woman with acupuncture, stopped the bleeding and revived her. How did Dr Sun know the woman in the coffin was not dead yet? From the blood drops from the coffin Dr. Sun knew the woman was bleeding that meant in her body there is energy pushing the blood to circulate. In a dead body there is no energy and the blood will not circulate. Dr. Sun's knowledge and experience made him a very famous doctor in Chinese history.

I would like to reveal a heaven's secret here. The secret is every person after age 40 must be responsible for his or her own appearances. What does this mean? People are born with good looking, ordinary looking, and not so good looking. We believe children's appearances are due to genetic factors that they inherited their parents' looks. That is true but there is another factor affecting a person's original look, that is what he has done in the previous life time also affects his look in this life. Physiognomy is a very profound knowledge. In this world there are only a few people that can tell a person's fate by observing his appearance. Parents' genes plus karma (good and bad) that a person created in his previous life time are the two factors that define his original look of this life. Many people at a young age look like angels but unfortunately that appearance dies away so quickly. There are also some people who were born ordinary looking and as they getting older they become more attractive. After age 40 a person's appearance and his living conditions are brought about by the last 40 years of his life experiences.

According to Chinese medicine theory, all skin problems are related to the poor quality of the blood. Acne is caused by toxic heat in the blood. Wrinkles, dry skin, dull skin, and pale complexion are due to poor blood circulation or blood deficiency. Senile plaques are due to liver blood deficiency. In Chinese medicine the diagnosis of blood deficiency indicates the poor quality of the blood or insufficient quantity of blood, or both. The diagnosis of western medicine is made by the count of the blood cells. Sometimes when I tell some people that their problems are caused by blood deficiency, they will say "I just had my blood work done and my doctor said my blood is fine." This is because blood tests don't show the quality of each cell. You may have the correct number but if the cells are not in good health you still can have blood deficiency symptoms. For this reason Chinese medicine can diagnose a health problem much earlier than western medicine. When a test of western medicine shows something is wrong in most cases the patients already have serious problems. For people over 50 to have younger looking skin they must constantly use food therapy to replenish the blood. Health wise, if there is no adequate blood passing through the liver and the heart that can cause liver and heart diseases as well.

If you have oily skin when you wash your face you can add a little salt in the wash water to help remove grease and prevent acne.

If you have dry skin you can add a little honey in your wash water or add a little vinegar in the wash water to make skin smooth and firm. Keep doing this to keep younger looking.

If you spend a lot of time on the computer, add some green tea in the wash water, green tea has anti-radiation effect, and can make the skin delicate and shiny.

If you have dark spots on your face, and your eyes are so tired or aging causes upper eyelids dropping, use hot water fomentation on the face to promote blood circulation and to get amazing results in a few days.

Home Remedy for Dry Skin

Some women complain about dry skin and itching skin. People with skin cancer were told by their dermatologists that skin cancer is due to exposure to the Sun. According to Chinese medicine theory, dry skin, itching skin, and even skin cancer are due to the poor quality of blood, causing the skin lack of nourishment. The peel of citrus fruit containing vitamin P that has moistens skin and anti-aging effects. Put orange peel or lemon peel into a blender. Add a little rice wine to cover the peel and blend for 5 seconds. Put the paste in an old sock and tie the opening. Drop it in your bath tub while you are taking a bath. You can have a spa treatment at home. To keep younger looking skin, remember to use replenishing blood remedies to treat the cause.

What is the Cause of Gray Hair and Hair loss?

1. Genetic? There is nothing we can do to change our DNA but according to the theory of Chinese medicine hair condition is related to the condition of the kidneys. Keep black sesame seeds, Gou Qi berries, and walnuts in your diet to promote hair growth.

2. For women after giving birth and going through menopause can accelerate hair loss. Use food therapy to nourish blood to improve hair condition.

3. If gray hair and hair loss start early in life, which is happening among many college students now. You should check your life style. Eating too much fried

food or spicy food can cause heat in the blood that can lead to hair loss. Spending long hours in front of a computer and staying up late will consume blood. Without adequate blood moving up to nourish the head will cause dry eyes, weak vision, dry hair, losing hair, and poor memory. Stress or being frightened also can cause gray hair and hair loss.

4. If hair becomes dry, less shiny, brittle, and easy to break this could be caused by harsh chemical treatments. Try to use natural products.

5. Gray hair growing in the frontal area is caused by a digestive system disorder. Gray hair growing at both lateral sides is due to heat in the liver and the gallbladder. Gray hair growing at the occipital area is due to kidney deficiency. If a person has gray hair all over his head, most likely he is smart and worries more, and easy to lose his or her temper. Try to be simple. The truth is life will be complicated for a person with a complicated mind. Nowadays human's mind has become more complicated and lead to the complication of human diseases.

Remedy for Dry Hair and Hair Loss

This remedy can be used for dry hair and losing hair caused by low energy and blood deficiency. Boil 15 grams of Gou Qi berries and 5 slices of fresh ginger in one liter of water for 10 minutes. Remove the Gou Qi berries and the ginger, and use the decoction to wash hair. Or store the decoction in a spray bottle and use as leave in conditioner. Keep the bottle in a refrigerator. Black sesame seeds and walnuts contain a large number of vitamin B group and vitamin E. Add them in your diet to nourish the kidney's essence and the blood, moisturize hair and promote hair growth.

Remedy for Gray Hair

Blood heat can cause hair loss and gray hair at a young age. Eat more multi-grains, celery, broccoli, cauliflower, carrot, walnuts, and pine nuts and avoid spicy food to improve the condition. Gray hair can give a person an older look. For both young and old with gray hair try this home remedy to turn the hair darker.

Ingredients: 250 grams of walnuts, 500 grams of peanuts with red skin, one bottle of vinegar

Soak the peanuts and the walnuts in the vinegar for one week. Everyday eat 5 peanuts and 3 pieces of walnuts for one month.

Or soak 100 grams of black beans in cold water over night. Cook the soaked black beans and 30 grams of walnuts in boiling water for 20 minutes. After the remedy cools down store it in refrigerator. Every day take 30 grams of the remedy and add 15 Gou Qi berries, and heat it up. Eat once a day to see improvement in a few weeks.

Another remedy works for Seborrheic hair loss, after illness hair loss, and postpartum hair loss.

Soak 500g of black beans in cold water for 2 hours. Put the black beans in a pot and add water just to cover the beans. Cook the black beans over high heat. When water is boiling change to low heat until the water is dried up. Spread the black beans on a big platter to let them dry. Sprinkle a little salt over the beans. After the beans dried store them in a glass jar. Eat the black beans twice a day and each time eat 25g of the beans.

Natural Hair Care

Add some vinegar or lemon juice in water at 1:10 proportion. Use the water to wash hair to reduce broken hair and make hair soft. For dry hair use milk to wash the hair and leave the milk on the hair, let the hair dry, then wash it with clean water. Although the smell is unpleasant the moisturizing effect is fantastic.

First add 1/8 bottle of beer in a spray bottle. Wash the hair clean and dry the hair with a towel. Evenly spray the beer all over the head. Gently massage the hair and the scalp for a few minutes. Leave the beer in the hair for 15 minutes then wash the hair with clean water. This beer therapy can promote hair growth and stop hair loss. Long-term use of beer massage can change the hair color to natural yellow and shine.

When cook rice save the water that was used to wash rice. Keep the water at room temperature for 1 to 2 days. Use the water to wash hair and use a tower to wrap the hair for

20 minutes. Then wash the hair with clean water. Washing hair with rice water often can make hair color darker and make the hair thicker.

For serious hair loss add 15g of salt in 1500ml of warm water and use the water to wash hair. The salt water can prevent and stop hair loss.

Remedy for Weight Loss

Nowadays people are very conscious about their weight and weight loss is a huge market. Many people come to see me say "I have tried all weight loss programs. No one really works." Most weight loss programs focus on the numbers not the people's health. What is the real cause of Obesity? Doctors, health care professionals and obese people themselves all believe an obese person's body is packed with fat. According to Chinese medicine theory and my own experience nine out of ten obese people are Qi deficiency (low energy) and have water retention in their bodies. Those fat people are like big water balloons, but the good news is to lose water is much easier and faster than losing fat. Blood and body fluid circulation rely on good energy. Good energy comes from strong metabolism. To protect your metabolic system you must avoid:

1. Unhealthy eating habits. Many people eat whenever they want, sometimes starving and sometimes overeating. Skipping meals to lose weight is a very wrong approach. Based on scientific study when a

person is in a state without food and drinks his digestive system, which includes organs like the stomach, liver, and gallbladder will secrete digestive juices as usual. If the digestive juices do not combine with food for metabolism but are absorbed by the body they will become toxic.

2. Prescription drugs are a big factor in making people gain weight. The major side effect of prescription drugs is damaging the metabolic system and causing water retention.

Remedy for Weight Loss

Ingredients: 100 grams of Chi Xiao Dou (Chinese red beans), 100 grams of mung beans (Chinese green beans), 30 grams of dried Shan zha (Hawthorn fruit), 10 dried dates

Soak the red beans and the Mung beans in cold water for one hour. Cook dried Shan Zha in 1000ml boiling water for 15 minutes, then remove the Shan Zha from the water and add the red beans, the Mung beans, and the dates to the Shan Zha decoction. Cook for 30 to 40 minutes. Drink the decoction and eat the ingredients every day. You can lose 10 pounds in two weeks.

Remedy to Brighten Eyes

I was told that if you keep using this remedy for 2 to 3 months you can throw away your reading glasses and have younger looking skin. I had perfect vision until I reached the age of 53. It is difficult for me to get used to wearing reading glasses. When I put on a pair of reading glasses I see myself immediately looking like a grandma. I tried this remedy and expected the results that I was told. After using this remedy less than one week I was surprised to see the prominent veins on my hands disappear. That is the sign of my blood circulation improving and the veins are softened. My eyes feel less tired even though I still need reading glasses but I feel much better. I spend a lot of time working on the computer and I am very happy with the result.

The amount of ingredients is for one person: ½ of a small potato peeled, ¼ of an apple peeled, ½ of a small tomato, Part of a carrot about 2 inches long

Cut all ingredients into small pieces and together put them in a blender, add some water to just cover the ingredients. Blend for 20 to 30 seconds and drink the whole thing before breakfast.

For night-blindness and vision loss, cook a small handful of black beans in boiling water for 15 minutes. Turn off the heat. Add in some Chrysanthemum and use the decoction to steam the eyes. Meanwhile use 6 grams of Gou Qi berries and 6 grams of Chrysanthemum to make tea. Use these two remedies every day to get the result quickly.

After some people read this book a question is raised. If all diseases can be cured, will people live forever? People will not live forever but no one has to die from a disease. If a person keeps himself in good health he will die a natural death. What is natural death? When the time is coming the person will be aware of it and prepared to go through the transition without any suffering. Unfortunately in this world 95% of people die of illness and only 5% of people die of natural death. Life is so precious. Take good care of yourself and your loved ones.

About the Author

I would like to introduce myself to my readers. I was born and raised in China. I never liked school because I only wanted to learn what I wanted to know. In order to make a living I earned a master degree of Chinese medicine and a bachelor degree of health science. Since there is no PhD of Chinese medicine available I believe I have enough knowledge of Chinese medicine. I am not a doctor or an expert of a particular area of medicine. I do practice Chinese medicine on all three levels. People come to see me with all kinds of health issues and I help them to quit prescription drugs, avoid unnecessary surgeries, and make them healthy again with natural therapies. I love what I am doing and very grateful for what I can do.

For health wise I am very blessed. When I was growing up there was no family member suffering illness and it was very rare to see prescription drugs in our home. From my early childhood to adulthood and becoming a mother, whenever I had health concerns I always seek two women's help, my grandma and my nanny not my parents. My parents are well-educated and well-traveled if they know I have health issues what they do is to take me to a hospital. My grandma and my nanny never got a chance to go to school. They cannot read or write. They never take me to hospitals. They use their way taking care of me. I remember when I was seven. One day I was with my nanny and suddenly I lost my vision. I shouted I cannot see. Nanny let me lied down in the bed on my stomach and did something on my back and also pressed one point on my hands. Less than ten minutes I got up and my vision was back to normal. Where we live is only two blocks away from a famous park in Beijing called Temple of heaven. Every morning my grandma and my nanny started their day by walking in that park. When I got pregnant grandma always came back from the park with some yellow pollen that she collected from Cypress trees. After my son was born grandma showed me to use the pollen as baby powder. Until I studied Chinese medicine I realized the pollen of Cypress is the best natural baby powder because the Cypress pollen has the therapeutic effect of clearing dampness and heat. Use it as baby powder can prevent diaper rash.

Cypress tree's Botanical name is Biota, and its leaves and seeds are used as herbs in Chinese medicine. The therapeutic effects of the leaf of Biota includes cooling the blood and stopping bleeding, stops coughing and expels phlegm, and promotes healing of burns. For early stage of burns grind the Biota leaves to powder and use the powder topically. You also can use Biota leaves to promote hair growth. After soaking the Biota leaves in a bottle of alcohol for one week, apply the alcohol on the scalp and massage a few minutes. It works.

In 1988 I came to the United States. In this country I was surprised to see many healthy people taking pills, later I learned those pills are vitamins. Another thing surprised me was when I heard people say "I have an appointment with my doctor." I was wondering "Wow in this country people have their own doctors." More than 25 years passed I still don't have a doctor. All these years I don't have health insurance, no doctor's visits except the dentist. The only one medical record I have is a free blood test I took at a health fair. In the year 2015 in order to avoid penalty I applied for Obama care but I have no intention to use it. It is not that I am invincible to all health issues. I went through so many stressful and painful experiences that helped me master powerful knowledge – natural healing. Like other immigrants I came to the United States alone with empty hands. I worked on different jobs and worried how to survive. In the past I experienced severe stomach pain, lower back pain, high blood pressure, high cholesterol, panic attack, etc., I had no money to see a doctor and actually I never thought about going to see a doctor. Whenever I had problem I would figure out what is wrong and went to a Chinese supermarket looking for herbal remedies or using food therapy, or spiritual healing and all worked well. In recent years, I don't have those health issues anymore, for taking care of myself I focus on maintaining good health and slowing down aging. With this book you can take good care of yourself, too. By the way, I taught myself English. Please forgive my mistakes in my writing. The desire that made me write is wishing everyone excellent Health.

Gina Yang

Cover Art by Ye Yuan

Editor: Lisa Garcia

www.naturaltherapywebsite.com

Email: ginayang@yahoo.com

Phone: 786-573-0553

ISBN: 9780692580035

Made in the USA
San Bernardino, CA
20 March 2016